Lily, Be Free

A True Account of Healing from Schizophrenia

by
Talitha Day Fair, Ph.D.

God's Chink-Filler Publications

2017

Acknowledgement

For technical assistance and encouragement on the original manuscript, thank you to:
Lowell E Becker, M.D.
Cornelia B. Wilbur, M.D. PSC

Dedication

To my mother, for her support and encouragement.
Without her, this story could not have been written.

CONTENTS

Preface
Chapter 1: Finding Out
Chapter 2: Removing Pressures
Chapter 3: Shoving Against the Walls
Chapter 4: Return to Purgatory
Chapter 5: Asserting Independence
Chapter 6: Guilt Confronted: Guilt Forgiven
Chapter 7: A Volcano, a Tunnel, and an Island
Chapter 8: Dr. Willoughby
Chapter 9: The Ward
Chapter 10: Forced Entry
Chapter 11: The Rock Takes Charge
Chapter 12: Forbidden Land
Chapter 13: Fire-Rain
Chapter 14: The Decision
Chapter 15: The Eruption
Chapter 16: Moving the Mountain
Chapter 17: The University
Chapter 18: Limbo
Chapter 19: The Crash
Chapter 20: First Encounter
Chapter 21: Worlds in Collision
Chapter 22: I'm Different
Chapter 23: Sickness, Not Uselessness
Chapter 24: Growing Up
Chapter 25: Trust Restored
Chapter 26: Thank God, I'm Schizie
Chapter 27: The Meaning of Suffering
Chapter 28: Salvation in This World
Chapter 29: Freedom

Author's Preface

If you had met Lily Farmer on the street of the southern college town in the 1960's, she would have smiled and greeted you politely; nothing in her polished façade would have betrayed that this model student was mentally ill. Diagnosed by the college psychologist as schizophrenic in her sophomore year, Lily fought for eight years to gain victory over the disease. What she learned in the struggle is relevant not only to persons with serious mental illness but also to individuals seeking to overcome inner conflicts that block their emotional and spiritual freedom.

When I first wrote Lily's story, (<u>Lily</u>, Accent Publications, 1982), I worked directly from her journals and case notes, staying as close as possible to the way events and counseling sessions actually occurred. But because real life does not arrange itself neatly into a story, that original manuscript was sometimes difficult reading. Therefore, the current retelling of the story is done more in the literary spirit of our time, with minor rearrangements in the sequence of events and elaboration of details to help the reader experience the world through Lily's eyes, while maintaining the integrity of the story. Names of people and identifying information have been changed, but terms used in the 1960's have been maintained, though some would be frowned upon today.

Psychology and psychiatry have changed in the past forty years, and it is because of some of those changes that Lily's story is important now. Currently, clinicians too often assume that schizophrenia and other serious mental illnesses are permanent and will always control the patient's life. So they hand out pills and provide some environmental support, rather than seeking to resolve the internal distress and bring about true healing. Even in cases of ordinary anxiety and depression, the goal of treating psychological and spiritual causes is frequently replaced with administration of mood-altering drugs, leaving the patient with the same problems and no improved skills for solving them.

Lily's story illustrates the possibility for the healing of major mental illness through psychotherapy, supported by biological treatment. It also provides principles that can guide counselors and individuals striving for psychological and spiritual wholeness.

Some readers may wonder if Lily's healing lasted and if she still would say that her illness had meaning. The answers are "yes". For thirty –five years, the woman referred to as "Lily Farmer" has been free of schizophrenic symptoms. She has enjoyed applying what she learned during her battle in a variety of settings-- home missions, the university psychology program where she earned her doctoral degree, and her own counseling practice. I know Lily continues to say, "Thank God for what I learned through being schizie."

I know for I am Lily.

CHAPTER 1– FINDING OUT
April 1966

The dismissal bell rang in the old Psychology/Education Building, releasing a noisy crowd of college students from the last class of the day. As they poured out through the double doors and into the Southern spring sunshine, Lily Farmer struggled toward the building, pushing against the flow, ignoring the cheerful greetings of friends. As she started up the cracked concrete steps at the entrance, she felt a tug on her arm.

"Hey, Lily, wait a minute," a voice shrilled from behind her. Lily turned to see a tiny freshman girl with a babyish face grinning at her. "Thanks for talking to me yesterday. I've decided to stay in college because of what you said. Now can you help me with my English comp paper so I can pass? Tonight, maybe?"

Lily smiled vaguely, staring into space over the girl's shoulder. "Not tonight. Hmmm, let's see. Tomorrow morning? 8:00 o'clock? Library? See you then."

Without waiting for a reply, Lily hurried into the building and through the dimly lit hallway. She climbed the creaking stairs leading to the second floor and collided head on at the top of them with a shapely senior in a pink mohair sweater.

"Ow! Watch where you are …Oh, it's you, Lily. I might have known," the senior grumbled. Then taking a more friendly tone, she said, "I needed to talk to you anyway. Would you do me a favor? I managed to get permission for an off-campus date this Friday. Would you substitute for me and play the piano for Women's Service League that night? Pleee-ase?"

Lily thought quickly. She enjoyed playing the

piano, but would her vision hold up for the late night meeting? Probably, if she rested during the afternoon. "All right, I'll do it. Leave the song book on the piano so I can practice."

"Thanks. You're an angel," the senior called, running down the stairs.

"Sure, just ask Lily. She can do anything. She always does," the sophomore muttered to herself as she stepped into the alcove leading to the door marked *Professor Leon Filbert*. She glanced at her Bulova watch. Seven minutes until time for her appointment. Too early. Lily leaned against the wall, smoothed the pleats in her green shirtwaist dress, and patted down her short chestnut curls. She pasted a smile in place and hoped that, to passing students, she appeared to be just another psychology major reporting for a routine conference. *Appearances are deceiving,* thought Lily. *And it's a good thing. How horrible if they knew why I am here.*

Involuntarily, her slim, muscular body tensed. Her breathing quickened. Her mind anticipated the impending battle. *I must win this fight. I must have the truth from him, and he must not see me flinch. Then we shall see what will be my doom.* Gathering all her will power, Lily knocked on the door, then stepped back, and watched the gold letters on the nameplate dance up and down. *Not now,* her inner monitor warned her. *Be calm, Lily. Smile, Lily. Don't let him see what is happening, Lily.*

The door rasped open and Lily Farmer looked straight at the tall, imposing man in the gray tweed suit and smiled mechanically. From behind her carefully constructed mask of calmness, she heard the psychologist's voice, gentle but compelling. "Lily, I'm glad you came. Come in and sit down."

Lily glanced around the sparsely furnished room, checking for any possible threat. Satisfied, she seated herself in the wooden armchair directly in front of the scarred oak desk. Arranging her limbs in what she hoped was a relaxed pose, she watched the professor take his seat behind the desk and pull from under the blotter pad a manila folder marked *Lily Farmer.* In spite of her determination to stay rational, she felt the room begin to sway.

Professor Filbert leaned forward, observing her intently. "How have you been feeling?"

The world spun. The varnished floor rose toward Lily, tilting her back, back into oblivion. "I—I," she stammered, and then was silent. It was upon her again—this thing, this monstrous force that had driven Lily, the model child, the star pupil, to the office of a psychologist. *Fight it,* she commanded herself silently. *You must stay rational. Fight.* She bit her lower lip hard.

"Lily, look at me," the psychologist ordered.

Lily forced her gaze upward from the treacherous floor until her smoldering green eyes met the professor's and were caught and held against her will. He was stronger than she, and from his steel gray eyes flowed a current that strengthened and empowered, a force that anchored Lily to reality. She had not wanted his power and yet, as her mind steadied a bit, she found she was grateful for it. But gratitude was dangerous and she must answer him as if nothing had happened.

"Prof, I've had kind of a hard time since you gave me those tests. But I can handle it. I have before. Would you please tell me what the tests showed?"

"Not so fast, Lily. Slow down and relax," he said, fingering the papers in her folder. "We have a whole hour; we don't need to hurry. I want to get to know you a little better. When you came in last week, you were pretty upset but you couldn't tell me why. Is there anything you want to tell me now?"

"Just that I'm having a difficult time thinking clearly. I keep forgetting where I am going and where I've been. Yesterday afternoon at 4:00 I woke up on my bed in the dorm. I thought I'd missed my classes, but when I got out my notebook, it had notes from my 1:00 and 2:00 o'clock lectures. I'd been there; I just couldn't remember them. Now that's a little scary."

Lily laughed nervously. "My roommate, Rebecca, says I've been acting strangely, talking to myself more, answering questions she didn't ask, staring into space. I told her I went through this in tenth grade and I worked it out myself. But, Prof, I would appreciate some help." Lily laughed again, fending off the cry of desperation that forced itself toward her lips. She must not show too much feeling; that was certain rejection.

"Lily, how do you get along with your parents?"

"Oh, my parents love me. I'm their only child and their whole lives revolve around me."

"But how do *you* feel about them?"

The power of the question sent Lily reeling through inner space. She searched her memory for a standard answer that would not reveal the emotions propelling her backward at a terrifying rate, away from the professor. She managed to say, "I love and obey them. I am a Christian, you know, and the Bible says to honor your father and mother."

"Lily, I can't help you unless you are honest with me."

The widening chasm between Lily and the psychologist filled with a white mist. Lily stared into the mist, searching for the strength of those piercing gray eyes.

"What do you do when you are angry?"

The voice led her to the eyes and she drew enough reality to answer. "I don't get angry. G—good Christians don't get angry." The white mist turned to a cottony fog that filled her mouth and throat.

"But you are angry," Professor Filbert insisted, seemingly unaware of the fog. "Intensely angry—with yourself, your parents, perhaps even with God. What do you do with your anger?"

"Nothing."

The fog choked her voice and seeped into her mind. *You're losing him; he'll be swallowed up into the fog in a minute. Fight, Lily, fight the fog.* Lily gripped the wooden chair arms, pulling herself forward toward reality.

Through the mist she could hear Prof Filbert calling her. "Lily, Lily, listen to me. Things in your life, now or in the past, maybe in your family, are upsetting you. You must tell me about them. We must face the hurt and get rid of the hostility."

Hostility—hostile—that word she understood. No one had ever told Lily it was a sin to be hostile, only to be angry. Her high school journals were full of the word *hostile*. The fog disappeared. The chasm closed. The cotton in her mouth came unstuck. Words revealing a few of the bitter experiences of the past twenty years rolled involuntarily from her mouth. After the words had ceased, Lily cringed, expecting the familiar authoritarian phrases of judgment and condemnation.

Instead, Lily heard, "It's all right for you to feel hurt and confused. It's natural and normal. But your parents and these other people did not mean to hurt you. Remember what Jesus said from the cross, 'Father, forgive them for they know not what they do.' Forgive your parents, teachers, and preachers. They meant well."

"I don't know how. I've said the words, 'I forgive,' but nothing ever changes."

"There are four reasons why people can't forgive," Professor Filbert explained, resorting to an academic approach. "They don't believe the other person is worthy of forgiveness. Or they are exalting themselves self-righteously. Or they equate forgiveness with condoning—saying the other guy is right. Or they want to make the other person suffer enough before forgiving him."

The words dropped around Lily as meaninglessly as tiny beads from a broken necklace clicking to the floor. "I don't know. I guess I fit all four categories. I usually do."

Though the words had been meaningless, Lily had drawn enough strength from their giver to feel more in control. The all-encompassing question must be asked and, with the fog gone and her mind clearer, this was the ideal moment. Lily smiled and with feigned casualness inquired,

"Prof, did you find out about the hostility from the tests I took last week?"

"Yes."

"What else did you find out?"

"Well, maybe we should discuss that another time."

"No, I want to know now. I can take anything as long as it is the truth."

Professor Filbert sighed, leaned backwards in his rickety swivel chair, and knit his bushy eyebrows. "All right. You have an unusually high degree of hostility. You live a good bit in fantasy. You have a depression score that is high, but lower than the other two. You are confused about your sexual identity."

"In other words, the same pattern we studied in class last week?"

"What do you mean?" he asked with a slight edge to his voice.

"Didn't we study a syndrome like mine in class? What do you think finally precipitated my seeing you?"

The psychologist paused, sighed as if making an uncomfortable decision, and then said, "I would like to circumvent that question, but from your being in my classes, I know how you function. If I don't tell you, you'll read and research until you find out anyway; then you won't trust me." Lily nodded in agreement. "So I may as well tell you. Your tests and emotional and behavioral symptoms are indicative of schizophrenia."

"In plain English, please."

"You have a form of schizophrenia."

"Thank you. I am then legitimate." The professor looked at her questioningly. "I can quit telling myself I have no right to experience the things I hear, see, and feel. I am legitimate. I am not making them up. Well, what shall we do about it? Do you think I'm going to totally break with reality?"

"Do you?" Professor Filbert asked, baffled at Lily's calmness. He was not accustomed to being cornered into giving a diagnosis, and he was certainly not accustomed to a client approaching her own disturbance so methodically.

"No, I've been this far out before."

"Well, I want to see you every week. If you need me between sessions, you can see me after class. We need to take off the immediate pressure. We'll see how you are in a couple of weeks. Then we will decide on the next step. Do you get along well with your roommate?"

"Oh, yes, Becca understands me. She has wanted me to get counseling."

"Do you have any tests in the near future?"

"Just in your class, and I'm ready for that."

"Then go back to your dorm and relax tonight. Let your studies go for a while."

In that hour, Lily Farmer had consciously and intentionally committed herself to the world of psychotherapy, determined not to relinquish it until she was free from her inner turmoil. With naïve trust, she pictured herself crossing the graduation stage, diploma in hand, free to greet the world.

CHAPTER 2—REMOVING PRESSURES
April 26, 1966

The morning after her self-commitment to psychotherapy, Lily turned over in bed and opened her eyes. Stifling a scream, she jerked the covers over her head.

"What's eating you?" her drowsy roommate grumbled from her bed on the opposite side of the room.

"Rebecca, help me! I saw you standing over me with a paring knife. You were going to kill me. Becca, it wasn't a dream!"

Rebecca Slone sat straight up. "Good grief, you are getting way out." She paused, and then added seriously, "Have you had any other hallucinations?"

"Last night I heard my grandmother calling me. I couldn't go to sleep because I was afraid she would hurt me."

"But, Lily, your grandmother is dead, and she was a nice lady," Rebecca said as she pulled her oversized body out of bed, flipped her dishwater blonde hair out of her eyes, and stared down at her friend.

"I know. Maybe I'm crazier than I thought I was."

"No. I think its just symptoms, but you'd better tell Prof Filbert anyway. And this afternoon after classes, let's go for a walk. Maybe getting off this campus will clear your head."

That afternoon when Lily returned to the dorm room, she found Rebecca sitting cross-legged on her bed, clipping magazine pictures for an assignment in Christian Education class. Although usually she would have been quiet when her roommate was working, Lily started talking rapidly--about spilling her test tube of gooey stuff all over her chemistry lab partner; about a freshman at her table in zoology lab stabbing their dissection specimen the wrong way and squirting formaldehyde in the professor's face;

about a friend's troubles with a boyfriend; and other bits of college trivia. But the more Lily talked, the more Becca concentrated on cutting up magazines and avoided looking at her.

Lily was perplexed: what was wrong with her roommate? Finally she said, "Let's get out of here."

Rebecca snapped, "The way you are acting, I'm not about to go off campus with you."

Wounded and confused, Lily fled the room.

Bewildered, Lily trudged off alone. Following a rut-filled dirt lane, she left the college and its surrounding village and wandered with her hurt through the low, rolling hills. Girls were not allowed off campus without special permission, but Lily's need to be alone often outweighed her habitual obedience to rules. This afternoon she had to escape the campus.

I can't let them see me crying, she thought. *I'm supposed to be a spiritual leader, and leaders don't cry. Especially in this town. We must be joyful all the time.*

But Lily couldn't choke back the tears of confusion. Why was Rebecca upset with her? Why wouldn't she go for a walk? What had Lily done? She just didn't understand. But recently there were so many things she did not understand.

Lily wandered along the familiar road until nearly suppertime, seeking the solace she usually found in nature. A fresh breeze ruffled her blue pleated skirt and teased her dark curls. Birds in the bushes sang their spring songs. Thoroughbred colts capered in the green fields. But today nature's beauty did nothing to ease her distress. Eventually she gave up and returned to the dormitory, hoping that her roommate would go with her to supper as usual. But Becca was not in their room. Instead, on her desk, Lily saw a note telling her to meet Rebecca at their special refuge, the college church in the center of town.

Lily found her roommate kneeling at the altar rail, staring upward at the stained-glass window that dominated the modern, white-walled sanctuary. Quietly Lily knelt beside Rebecca. "Whatever I did, I'm sorry. Why are you mad at me?"

"Mad at you?" Rebecca's pudgy face was streaked with tears, but her voice was steady and soothing. " I thought you were upset with me, Lily. I just couldn't take any more from you. I figured you would have calmed down by now."

Lily gave Rebecca a look that meant, "Uh-oh," then said, "Uh, Becca, did I get confused again or something?"

"I'm not sure. Maybe it was just a misunderstanding. You've acted so weird lately that I don't know for sure. Yesterday at the drugstore lunch counter I said I didn't like chocolate malts. Five minutes later you said you didn't like chocolate malts and you used my identical words. But Lily, you *love* chocolate malts."

"Becca, sometimes I forget whether I'm me or you. In class, sometimes I think I'm the prof. I catch myself asking him the question he just asked me. It's like I switch roles with the other person; I'm he and he is me. Would you say I have an identity problem?"

"Slightly!" Rebecca stood up. "Come on; let's walk out to the haunted house. It can't be any spookier than this conversation."

That weekend, Lily spent most of her time curled up in a corner of her bed, her back against the dingy yellow wall. At first, she propped a book on her knees to give the appearance of studying, but she and Rebecca both knew it was a sham. Lily had simply withdrawn. For forty-eight hours, Lily lived in a numbness of nothingness, rejoining the college world only when Rebecca used special words and a particular grasp on Lily's arm, what Lily called "The Keys to the Kingdom". Becca used the " Keys" to force her friend to emerge from the cocoon for meals, exercise, and sleep. She left church and social activities to Lily's choice, and Lily blocked out the world.

May, 1966

Tuesday, when Lily arrived for her appointment

with Professor Filbert, her inertia was breaking into histrionics. "From catatonia to mania," she mumbled as she mounted the worn wooden stairs.

To her dismay, the psychologist's office door was locked. She leaned against the faded yellow wall and waited, trying to appear casual, unconcerned. But the inner accusations could not be silenced. *He really doesn't care. He just wanted enough information to condemn you as crazy. He'll ignore you now. Wait and see.* Lily felt her carefully constructed, smiling mask slipping.

To her horror, another psychology professor who was passing in the hall stopped and surveyed her questioningly. "Are you waiting for Professor Filbert? He will be in a committee meeting all afternoon."

Lily stammered a "thank you" and dashed down the steps to hide her tears and her ragged breaths. As she staggered toward her dorm, a dense fog settled over her mind. Prof had not even bothered to leave her a note. He really didn't care. He was making a game of her. Nothing mattered now, *nothing.*

That evening, rest and rationality eluded Lily. Though Rebecca had helped her to bed early, she did not sleep but drifted in and out between the real world and terrifying fantasies. About midnight, Lily's mind cleared enough for her to scrawl a note to the psychologist. "Prof, this torment is going to stop! Either I will deliberately withdraw or I will--."

She had no intention of suicide, but she would rather it sounded that way than reveal her true thoughts of destruction—her visions of broken windows and burning books. Withdrawal would probably be her course. No one else would be hurt by withdrawal.

Early the next morning, Lily shoved the note under Professor Filbert's office door. She dragged through the day, extending an arm to balance on ground that felt like it slanted at a 45-degree angle. Lily had lab work to do in chemistry, and she silently pleaded with Jesus to clear away the mental mist enough for her to complete it. Somehow she finished the assignment—not well, but adequately.

With a fifteen-minute break before zoology lab, Lily struggled to the college post office. If Prof cared, he had had time to leave an answer to her note in her mailbox. If not, she would black out all awareness of reality and sit absolutely motionless right in the middle of zoology lab. Someone would have to do something. She really didn't care what, as long as the hopelessness stopped.

Lily opened her mailbox. There was a letter in Prof's precise handwriting! He did care! The notes said that yesterday he had left a message at the front desk in the dormitory; he was sorry that the message had not been given to her. He would see her at their regular time. Lily let out a deep sigh, smiled, and mechanically went through the form of living for the next two hours of class

At 5:00 p.m. Lily sat in the church in the second pew waiting for Rebecca to finish her counseling session with Pastor David. Her roommate also had been under a great deal of internal strain. Her family was disintegrating; Rebecca, never secure, was terrified of being abandoned. Bearing the weight of both Rebecca's problems and her own, Lily gazed upward toward the stained-glass window. The window was cut in the shape of a cross; yet, the Christ was not in agony but in the triumph of ascension, a cloud under his feet, his arms outstretched to greet the Heavens. Lily searched the face of the Christ for some comfort, some measure of assurance that, as He had conquered the grave and hell, she too would conquer this living death that was all she knew of life.

Oh, Jesus, she cried silently, *I love you. Deliver me from this inner torment. You, who are the Way and the Life, show me the path out into the world where those other students live, laughing, happy, and free. Make me free. Make Rebecca free.*

Lily waited, eyes fixed on the crystal figure. Always before when she had prayed in this church, from this second pew, watching the cross from this angle, there had been an answer, a faint glimmer of a smile and a tender softening in the face of the distant Christ. Perhaps the glimmer was only an alteration in the sunlight filtering through the colored glass: that did not matter to Lily. It was a sign, an answer, and that was all she asked. But today the light did not change; the face did not soften. There was only the cold, crystalline image staring into the beyond.

Oh, Jesus, can it be that You do not hear me? She paused as an idea occurred to her. *Or perhaps do I believe too strongly in the magic of the window? Give me some sign of Your love.*

At the left of the sanctuary, a door squeaked open. Glancing sideways, Lily saw Pastor David and Rebecca coming toward her, still deep in conversation. Pastor David's tender expression toward Becca reminded Lily of a grandfather comforting a young child who had just skinned her knee. A moment later the pair stopped beside Lily.

"Hello, Lily." Pastor David smiled at her and all of the light and tenderness she had hoped to see in the crystal Christ broke through on the pastor's face. "It's good that you are here." Because of the light, Lily felt that Pastor David truly wanted her here, in his church, and it felt strange to be wanted--strange but good.

"Rebecca tells me you girls have been sharing your problems with each other." Lily cringed, expecting the familiar people-shouldn't-talk-about-their-problems lecture. Instead she heard, "That's good. God knew that you both needed a friend who would understand, and He gave you to each other. Not many young people experience the kind of friendship you have. See you both on Sunday."

As Pastor David disappeared through the sanctuary door, Lily thought, *the light and the sign don't always come through magic and ritual; sometimes, maybe most of the time from now on, they come through people. I understand, Jesus.* Carefully she laid aside one of the rules that made her world different from other people's and took one tiny step into normality.

By Thursday, when Lily again met with Professor Filbert, the experience in the church had worn off. In its place, hallucinations, role exchanges, and other confusions were wrecking what little she knew of reality. But Lily was not in the habit of showing her true emotions. Seating herself in the battered wooden armchair across the desk from the psychologist, Lily forced her body into a relaxed position. With feigned casualness, she spoke of these terrifying distortions as though they were merely academic matters.

Unfortunately, Professor Filbert answered accordingly. "Don't worry about them. They are just symptoms. Your controls are low. It's like a hand trying to hold a dozen fishing corks under the water at once. Images—corks—keep popping up from your unconscious mind. There are more conflicts than you can hold down at once." Lily nodded that she understood. "How are your grades?"

"Not good. I'm getting B's in my two science classes. That won't do if I am to get into medical school. Lab work is terribly hard for me now, even with the best professor in the department. Frankly, I'm scared to death about taking organic chemistry next year with Dr. Mole. He talks way over my head, and he speaks so softly I can't understand him."

"Doctor who?" Filbert questioned sharply.

"Oh, I'm sorry!" Lily stared at a crack in the floor as her face reddened. "You know what's-his-face. Mole is my name for him; I give many people animal names. It just slipped. I didn't mean to be disrespectful."

The psychologist chuckled at Lily's characterization of that pointed-nosed, hunched-back teacher, habitually dressed in moleskin brown. "That's all right," Prof Filbert reassured, watching for a reaction from Lily, a reaction that did not come. The psychologist did not yet know that the stronger Lily reacted internally, the less she showed on the outside.

Unable to see Lily's profound relief created by his lack of condemnation, Prof Filbert changed the subject. "Back to the issue of classes. Perhaps you should put away the idea of medical school for a while. Not competing for A's would relieve part of the immediate pressure."

Lily swallowed hard. For five years she had planned to go to medical school. She was taking a double major in zoology and psychology to be well prepared. She wanted to help people, it was true, but she also wanted to show all those public school teachers whom she had resented that she could be a great intellect. Their mediocrity and criticalness could not hold her back! However, since she saw the psychologist's point and had no logical response that would not betray her emotions, she said, "I guess you are right. Maybe I can find some easier career in biology, something that wouldn't require organic chemistry."

The professor pulled out a pamphlet on medical careers. "Maybe physical therapy would interest you. Read this. I think you would be good in a children's hospital.

Lily smiled. At least Prof didn't think she was totally useless.

"Lily, as you let go of some of the present stressors, we can begin to get to the root of your disturbance. I've been wondering how far back these problems extend. When do you think they began?"

"I'm not sure," Lily hedged. She was quite sure of the birth date of her fantasy world, but that world she must conceal at all costs. As to the other problems, all life was a problem.

"You mentioned last session that you had similar symptoms in tenth grade. Would you tell me what happened then?"

Lily stared at the rough floorboards, torn between the potential relief of self-revelation and the fear of its consequences. "I'm not sure I can explain it calmly."

"Lily, it's safe to get upset in here. I'll help you handle your feelings. Look at me."

Once again Lily locked her green eyes into the psychologist's silver grey ones, drawing from his resources. Abruptly she turned away in shame. "Prof, I don't want you to think I was a bad kid. Most of my teachers thought I was a model student--bright, studious, and concerned about others, a bit over-conscientious maybe."

"Lily, you do not have to defend yourself to me."

"But I want you to know how people saw me. The problem was that they had no idea what was happening that they didn't see."

"What was that?" asked Professor Filbert, observing her with increasing concern.

"Like what happens now. I would be sitting quietly in class, trying to concentrate. Without warning, a tremendous force would swell up inside me, making me want to scream, to hit, and to run out of the room. I'd fight to sit still and smile on the outside. But I could feel myself mentally drifting backwards, until the class seemed miles away and I could barely hear the teacher. I think the technical word is withdrawal. Eventually I learned to withdraw at will to control the pressure, but when I withdrew, I couldn't participate in class. I didn't like that. Anyway, withdrawal didn't always work. Often, by the time I got home from school, the pressure inside would be overwhelming. My mother didn't get home from teaching second grade for an hour after I did; so, blessedly, I was alone. That's when it would happen."

"What would happen?" Prof Filbert leaned forward and opened his hands in a gesture of concern.

"The explosion. I'd start yelling and crying and throwing things. Only it wasn't me. It was like something else had taken control of me. Somehow I never broke anything significant, and I always cleaned up the mess before Mother got home. No one ever saw—until *that* day." Lily stopped. Motionless, she stared at an invisible point on the wall behind the psychologist's head.

"What day?" the psychologist prompted.

"That day at school. At the end of my freshman year, my Latin teacher had promised me I could enter the state foreign language contest. I studied all summer, but when my sophomore year started, he wouldn't let me enter.

According to him, my class was progressing too slowly. I tried to tell him I knew all of the second year grammar and could read and understand *Caesar's Gaelic Wars* without translating it. But he wouldn't listen. I had loved and trusted him, but he turned out to be just like all the other teachers and preachers. He didn't care." Lily teetered on the edge of her chair, fingernails gouging into its arms, voice shrill with anger.

"Lily, relax. You were hurt and disappointed. Your feelings were normal."

"Yes, and for the first time in my life, I let my feelings show. I wouldn't speak to the teacher except when he asked me to translate. Then I'd read the Latin and give the meaning instead of a word-for-word translation. I was going to prove to him what I could do. I openly ignored the homework, but on tests I always got the highest grade in the class. Prof, I desperately longed for him to call me in and tell me he cared and wanted to help."

"But he never did?"

"No. Instead he gave me a 'B' on my report card. A "B" was one insult I couldn't tolerate. Internal pressure soared beyond control. I marched up to his desk and fairly screamed at him. How dare he cut my grade? He was jealous, stupid, and trying to get even. He was a liar as well. He was no teacher. He was a dunce, an egotistical idiot.

"Then I ran from the room and hid in a remote rest room. Since there was a pep rally the next period, no one missed me. While the cheerleaders beat on the drums, I beat on the metal partitions between the stalls until my hands were raw. I screamed; I cried. There was no relief. It was like a volcano erupting without end.

"Somewhere there had to be relief. I pulled out my notebook and started to write. Without realizing exactly what I was doing, I wrote that the way to stop the pain was to stop feeling. Therefore, I would no longer feel. I would split my personality in half. One half of me would think and the other half would feel. The thinking half would function when I was in public and the feeling half only when I was alone."

Deliberately, Lily did not mention that the "thinking half" had incorporated another self, one whom she had previously called "imaginary". On that day, this other identity, an invincible girl from another world, had become a part of her.

"I walked out of the restroom and joined the lunch line, calm, cool, collected, as though nothing had happened. I had solved the problem of feeling. I could control the pressure and still function academically and socially."

By this time, Lily was sitting back in her chair in relaxed dignity, as though she were a queen speaking to a friend of lesser rank.

"And was escaping reality a satisfactory solution?" Professor Filbert leaned forward intently.

"Who's escaping?" she replied lightly. "I simply discovered a unique self that could survive."

"Lily, you are playing games with me and you know it. You know I can't let you go on with this. Now look squarely—"

Panic seized Lily. The psychologist was about to break through into a world she had secreted for years. A world that held the key to her survival. "To be exposed is to die," a voice deep within her warned. The room tilted chaotically; a chasm opened in front of the professor. She called out in terror, "Prof, please, please don't. I can't take it! I've got to stay in school. Don't pull me apart!"

"Easy, Lily. It's all right," he said, coming around the desk and standing close to her. Although the psychologist viewed Lily's explanation of her split more as avoidance of pain than as a reality ruling her existence, he knew that penetrating her defenses too quickly could precipitate a break with reality. He changed his tone to that of gentle support. "Relax. You are safe. Now take two deep breaths. That's right. You don't need to be afraid." He paused, making a mental note that this girl was much more fragile than she had wanted him to know. He must move slowly. "We'll go at your pace. We are in this together." Again he paused, observing her clinically. As Lily's breathing and skin coloration returned to normal, he reassured her, "You did very well to tell me so much today. You can always tell me just as much as you want to."

"Okay. And thanks." Lily leaned her tousled brown head back, relaxing her tense muscles. At least Prof Filbert could be trusted not to pry too deeply and not to condemn what he did not understand. The systematic part of her mind dictated that she must dim his memory of the clues she had given him to her innermost world.

"Prof, I want you to know that after my sophomore year in high school, things improved."

Seeing that Lily was ready to talk on her own, Professor Filbert returned to his chair. Resting his arms on his desk and picking up his pen, he nodded, encouraging her to keep talking. He wanted time so that Lily's defenses would be well in place and her controls strong before he brought up a painful current dilemma.

Lily continued. "I spent that summer at the university experimental high school taking chemistry. I loved university life—the quiet, the intellectual stimulation. The research in the term paper I wrote on the biochemistry of tranquilizers surprised me. The findings of my term paper also surprised my chemistry teacher and the university biochemistry professor. That success proved to me I could master any academic area if I could keep my mind clear. My mind was as bright and quick as the IQ tests had indicated. I felt a little better about myself.

"In my junior and senior years, I was in many activities—speech contests, class plays, student congress, church programs, girls' athletics, library and English club. I graduated salutatorian, well respected for my brains."

"I'm glad your life improved, Lily. That is a good sign that you can work through your problems now." The psychologist paused reflectively. "And I have to talk with you about a present problem that we must solve today," he said cautiously. He cleared his throat, obviously reluctant to approach the topic. "How much do your parents know about your psychological difficulties?"

"Very little. I never told them what was happening to me in high school, except that I was angry with the B in Latin. In the past, whenever I had confided in them, it shook their image of me as a model child, and they didn't know how to react." Lily tilted her head, an expression of pity on her face. "They can't accept any change in me. I have to live according to their preconceived image. For example, last spring during the college revival, I wrote home about some of the college's doctrines that were new to me, and about trying to decide if they were true. I said I was searching for a deeper spiritual life. My mother got upset and wrote to the Dean of Women, making a lot of accusations and not much sense. So now I tell my parents very little."

"We have to tell your parents that you are coming for counseling." He paused briefly, waiting for Lily's reaction. When she did not respond, he continued, " You have said you want to stay for summer school. Your parents have a right to know why. Also, they may be able to help you better understand your past."

Within Lily's head, a tumultuous storm of fear rumbled a warning. "They're not going to like the idea. They think I'm a perfect, loving, brilliant model-child. I better tell them myself."

"What if you write a letter and I write a letter? We'll compare them before we send them. Is that all right?"

"Yes, but please don't ever write to my parents without my knowledge. Odd things can happen." Lily did not notice that the psychologist had not answered her. The conversation drifted to trivia and finally ended.

Lily continued her twice-weekly therapy sessions. She asked dozens of academic-sounding questions—about symptoms; about the relationship of body, mind, and spirit; about the nature of therapy. The professor answered each question thoroughly while trying to discover the origin of the illness in this young woman from a seemingly normal background. Yet he never probed directly into her childhood, and Lily, though bursting with pain of those early years, never told him. She wanted solutions, change—not sympathy—and how could one change what had happened years ago?

On the Friday after her last semester examination, Lily talked with Professor Filbert about her parents' upcoming visit to meet with the psychologist. "How are you going to explain my sickness? They will not be happy about this. Make it as easy as possible for them."

"Your parents are Christians, right?"

Lily nodded.

"I want to explain the role of therapy from a Christian standpoint. For any event to occur—physical, mental, or spiritual—there must be both necessary and sufficient conditions. A car on a hill with the brake set has the necessary potential energy to go forward. But the brake interferes with the necessary conditions. If we apply this analogy to you, psychotherapy removes the brakes—those unhealthy things deep within you—so that the conditions of health already present can operate. God has provided the sufficient conditions. I Corinthians says, 'My grace is sufficient for thee.'"

"That sounds good," Lily responded quickly, too quickly, covering up her true thoughts. She did not agree that health was already in her, but her parents would like the analogy.

On Saturday, Mr. and Mrs. Farmer arrived on campus and conferred with Professor Filbert. The Farmers agreed that Lily could attend summer school. Though they were shocked that their daughter had psychological difficulties, they seemed eager that she receive whatever treatment she might need. Professor Filbert assured them that Lily felt comfortable with him and that he expected her to improve. Without telling Lily, the psychologist promised to keep the Farmers informed concerning their daughter's progress.

Lily spent a week at home with her parents, and then returned for the summer term at college.

CHAPTER 3—SHOVING AGAINST THE WALLS
June 1966

Lily tackled the summer term as one continuous therapy session, utilizing her academic strength to devise her own plan for solving her problems. On the second day of summer school, she sat outdoors, her back against the trunk of a shady maple near the dormitory, writing in a spiral notebook. "I have decided it is important to keep a detailed journal of my experiences. A credible scientist does not trust her memory but records everything she observes about her subject. I am my own subject; therefore, I must record whatever I observe or learn about myself—my actions, my thoughts, my feelings. The writing may be factual or emotional, according to situation and content. Like a good scientist, I will review my records at intervals to look for patterns and to remind myself of what I have learned. I ask God's blessing on this journal."

When not in class, Lily haunted the library, reading all of its meager collection on schizophrenia and making copious notes. On June 17, she sat in the library. Though she was writing, her face was a study in blankness. "It's strange to see myself in print, or at least the odd parts of myself, as in a description in a textbook today. 'Afraid of self…seeks to control everything in environment…emotional blunting…distorts reality to meet own needs…unable to relate to people… depressed… hostile… lives in fantasy….' But I *must* read. If I know what I'm fighting, I can attack it better. I haven't mentioned my research to Prof. You know how these experts are. They don't think the patient should be informed, as if knowledge were infectious. But they don't have to deal with my turmoil 1,440 minutes a day, 10,080 minutes a week. They put in their sixty minutes and walk away. I have to live with me."

On June 20, as she sat on the dormitory steps, watching students playing Frisbee in the grassy semi-circle, she wrote, "I don't understand these college girls. They seem to think life is peaches and cream. My summer roommate's sweet, pure, healthy, happy disposition astounds me. How can anyone be so happy in this horrible world? She can't understand me either, but she is friendly to me. When I told her I am having mental problems and can't see to read sometimes, she said she would be glad to help me with my work. Yesterday she asked me to go bike riding with her and her friends. She didn't get angry when I was poky. Too bad she can't know the thrill of riding a bicycle when the road is flapping like a sheet in the breeze. It's quite a trip! Ha!

"Several of my old friends seem to know I am having problems and have offered to help 'because we like you.' I don't know why anyone would like me, but I appreciate the help."

June 21, alone at her desk in her room, Lily wrote: "Dear Jesus, Thank You for using me tonight. At least I am good for something. When I took on the job of leading our Christian service project at the state institution for delinquents, I was looking for a way to escape from my own problems for a few hours a week. I didn't think I could really help those teenagers. Why would they listen to a goody-two-shoes like me? But something special happened tonight. As I was talking to twelve-year-old Judi, who always wants my attention, the matron came over. She is usually a grouch and was certainly not a person I wanted to see right then. I already had a headache and upset stomach from being with people.

"Instead of griping as usual, the matron said, 'A girl named Joan wanted to talk to you earlier today, but she is in solitary now. Would you mind going up to see her?'

"I looked questioningly at Judi. 'Go, Miss Lily. Joan's is going to kill herself if someone doesn't stop her. She needs you worse than I do.'

" 'I'll go,' I told the matron. I was honored; volunteers are rarely permitted in solitary. But as I rode the ancient clanging elevator up to what the girls had dubbed 'The Tower,' I found myself wondering if this was really a trap. Was the matron watching for evidences of craziness in me so she could report me? Or worse, was this grinding metal cage taking me into another world inhabited by movie screen beasts? Was I doomed—?

"*Stop this nonsense!* I mentally ordered myself. *You must stay reasonable and responsible. God, hold me steady.*

"As the matron locked the door of the dirty, cramped isolation cell door behind me, I almost vomited. The cell contained only a cotton mattress and an open toilet: it reeked of anger, hate, and despair. Opposite me stood a scantily clad teenage girl, taller and more muscular than I. She had a raw gash across her cheek and rag bandages around her wrists. Nauseated, I wanted to mentally escape, to run to the protection of my fantasy world.

"*Do not run,* I ordered myself. *This girl needs you. Make her feel secure with you. Do for her what Prof Filbert does for you.*

" 'Hello, Joan,' I said, trying to sound calm and confident. 'I'm Lily from the college. You wanted to talk with me?'

"At first Joan glared and flexed her muscles. I thought she was going to flatten me with her fists. But within a half hour we were sitting side-by-side on the mattress on the floor, with Joan pouring out her hurts and fears. She had tried to kill herself once, and she would do it again and again until she succeeded if something didn't change, she said. I tried to say what I thought Prof Filbert would say, and, to my surprise, it worked. Joan calmed down. She made me promise to see her each week, and she promised to read the verses I marked in an easy-to-read New Testament.

"What an experience? Jesus, if I hadn't had my own

problems, I would never have known how to help Joan. Thank You for using my pain to help someone else."

Two days later, Lily wrote quite a different entry. " June 22, I have a new problem. A week ago, several of us went from sociology class to the cafeteria together for lunch, including Xavier, one of the three black students on campus. He is a prince in his tribe in Africa and has worked along side the medical missionaries from our college. Now he wants to attend an American medical school and then return to help his own people. We both argue a lot with the prof in sociology class. At lunch, Xavier sat down beside me at the long table. As the group's conversation turned away from us, Xavier said quietly, 'Miss Lily, you are a fascinating woman.'

"I turned pale: I didn't know what to do. No man had ever found me fascinating—certainly never African royalty. As we talked, Xavier said he feels isolated here and he rarely opens up to girls, but he shared with me about his country, his original home life, and his faith. We talked for an hour until the cafeteria closed.

"Why did he grant me such a privilege? I'm awkward, socially stupid, ugly, naïve. Xavier speaks eight languages, has a degree from Oxford, and is a cultured gentleman. When he looks at me, I'm walking on pink clouds. All my confusions vanish. Nothing could possibly be wrong when I'm with Xavier.

"Kind of hopeless, isn't it? I remind myself that this relationship can't go further. We aren't allowed to talk alone on campus because of the no-interracial-fraternization rule. And Xavier will be leaving soon. I tell myself not to get emotionally involved, but I don't listen very well. We have been meeting everyday in an out-of-the-way room in the library, supposedly to study sociology. But my interest is definitely not sociology, and I doubt that Xavier's is either."

Xavier continued to treat Lily with dignity and grace and tenderness, and Lily responded accordingly. On June 25, she wrote, "My feelings toward Xavier shatter the foundation of my old taboo against talking to boys. I expected that being with a man, just talking and caring, would doom me to something horrible. But knowing Xavier has made me stronger, almost happy at times. I wonder what would happen if I talked to other male students?"

July 1966

"I wondered and I found out," Lily wrote on July 2 as she relaxed on her bed, her journal on her lap. "What a day! During summer term, the college always plans a Saturday social event for us. We are all expected to attend. Today we all took a bus to a state park for a picnic, except for the three black students and a few others who had on-campus responsibilities. The park was beautiful—all green with wildflowers and great hills and valleys. But I was too spatially disoriented to enjoy it at first. A half hour after we got off the bus, I was still standing by the road, looking down a steep grassy hill at the couples strolling through the valley below. The clear river that had cut that valley twisted among the white rocks like a double silver chain. I wished I could sit beside its cool foam and dabble my feet in the water. But I knew that I couldn't navigate the terrible climb down: space was too capricious and the ground, too unpredictable.

"I was considering getting back on the bus when I heard a voice behind me. 'Hi, Lily, come down with us.' There was Lin, a mature Chinese gentleman here just for the summer, and with him was that tall, skinny freshman known as a religious fanatic. 'Don't be afraid. We will help you.' With formal courtesy, Lin took my hand to help me, and the freshman led the way down to the river.

"Having guys help me? I thought, as we climbed down the hill. *What kind of a sissy am I?* But they didn't think I was a sissy! I watched them carefully. They actually enjoyed helping me and having me with them! The afternoon slipped by as quickly as the twigs on the river. When we joined other picnickers at the tables for supper, I

laughed a lot, and the guys thought I was laughing at their jokes. But I was laughing at my old taboo, *Avoid men. They are dangerous.* Guys can be fun. What have I been missing all these years?"

By her next session with Professor Filbert, the charm of that afternoon had faded. After recounting the day's events, Lily said, "I enjoyed the attention. But something in my subconscious mind is nagging at me."

Swiveling back and forth in his desk chair, Prof grinned a boyish, unprofessional grin. "Are you afraid of your sexual feelings?"

"No, it's not that. I used to think sex was sinful, but Pastor David's class on Christian dating showed me that God wants us to enjoy our sexuality," Lily evaded quickly, not believing a word she said. "The problem in my head is deeper."

Lily watched her psychologist settle into listening mode; then she gazed at the picture in her mind of herself beside the river. "At the picnic, I felt so—so grown up." Abruptly her face contorted, as the pathology inside her took control. "That's it, Prof. Grown up. I must not grow up. It's too dangerous."

"What is dangerous?"

"I don't know. Just growing up." Lily pressed her left hand against her temple as if to hold her head in place. With the other hand, she held tightly to the chair arm to keep from feeling like she would drift upward out of her seat.

The psychologist leaned forward, probing intensely. "Are you violating one of those pet standards of yours again? Is there a standard, 'it's wrong to grow up' or 'It's wrong to enjoy myself'?"

"Both! Both! I mustn't! No! I won't be like those adults. I won't lie to kids. I won't condemn and misunderstand like they did. I won't torture children with promises, and then laugh at their hurt when the promises are broken. I won't!"

Professor Filbert asked sharply, "Do I hurt and

misunderstand and condemn?"

Lily paused. Her first inner response was, "Yes": he had recently expelled two of her college friends for having bad attitudes. But she did not know the whole story behind the expulsions, and Prof had been kind to her. "No, you've always been accepting of me," she said with more control.

"Am I an adult?"

"Yes."

"Where did your concept of adults come from?"

"Home."

"And?"

"School. Church. TV."

"General social experience and stories you heard, right?" Lily nodded in agreement. "For a girl who says she can't generalize in her class work, you certainly generalize about people."

Patient and psychologist laughed, and the laughter cleaned away the infection from old wounds inflicted upon her by too many adults in her past.

"Okay, I get the point," Lily said, leaning back in her chair. "I didn't realize I still pictured adults that way. You know, I used to sing a song about 'adults are kids gone sour'. Well, I guess I have a few decisions to make, don't I?"

"What?" The question startled the psychologist. Then, catching on to Lily's quick shift to problem-solving mode, he smiled and said more lightly, "Yes, I suppose you do."

"Stop grinning. Just because I'm crazy doesn't mean I'm stupid. I can think out a few things--but I suppose most crazy people don't plan their own therapy."

"No, they don't," Professor Filbert chuckled self-consciously. "And you're not crazy."

Pretending to ignore his comment, Lily cut in. "They don't plan their therapy because they don't know how. See, I have the advantage of your expert instruction in class."

The professor bowed teasingly.

"Seriously, I need a new picture of adults," Lily admitted. "I guess you and the dean's wife and Pastor David will do for patterns. Now my next question is, if I refuse to grow up, can I just stay the same?"

Frustrated yet amused that he had lost control of the session again, Prof Filbert sighed and explained in an academic tone, "No, you will inevitably regress. You have no chance of vocational success or of Christian witness. There is a law behind Paul's statement, 'Grow up in all things in Jesus Christ.'"

"It figures. Growing up is the lesser of two evils. Jesus had to grow up. I guess I can too." The decision made, Lily never turned back. She put a reminder card in her journal: *I must grow up: Jesus did.*

August 1966

For the remainder of the summer, Lily continued to shove relentlessly against the walls that locked her within her own being. Bit by bit she gained more freedom than she had ever known in her twenty years of life.

Lily's success with the Christian service project improved her feeling of self-worth. August 2nd, she wrote: "If the summer were otherwise worthless, the victories with the delinquent girls would vindicate its existence. During the summer, Judi understood who Jesus is and prayed for salvation. Whether she meant the prayer or was just trying to please me, she made one small, healthy step.

"Joan amazes me. She is calming down, is reasonable, calls me her big sister, and talks about hope and a future. It seems she needed the enforced quiet of isolation, a few people who cared, and physical protection. Her social worker is sufficiently impressed to have arranged for Joan to go live with a relative out of state. Saying good-bye tonight was hard for both of us. She says she'll never forget the neat, clean college girl who cared enough to sit on a stinking floor and hug her. I know I'll never forget the thrill of loving someone who knew only hate and then watching her gradually respond."

In contrast to her success in helping these teens, Lily was powerless against her own emotions that vacillated erratically within hours. On the final Sunday of summer school, Lily recorded their unpredictability in her journal. "August 7, 1966, 5:00 p.m. Xavier! Xavier! Being with him tonight at supper was being intensely alive. I'm sorry he is returning to Africa, but I will treasure the love and the respect I have known from him.

"8:00 p.m. Concerning church tonight. As the sanctuary lights dimmed, the stained glass cross in the front of the church glowed with life. Through the congregation swelled the old hymn 'Jesus Keep Me Near the Cross.' My heart rushed from this imprisoning body to be held and warmed and comforted by the Great Comforter. The Christ in the window, arms outstretched, embraced my soul. For one brief moment, I was Christ's, and He was mine.

"9:30 p.m. I cannot study. Tossing, I am tossing in the waves. High into the air, then under the sea. Waves of light crashing against me. Sinking, sinking. The sea is closing over me. I am under the sea. Thousands of pounds of water-light are pushing me down, down into extinction. I am crushed, smothered, dying. Help, God, help.

"Withdraw, withdraw to the Island. There, no one can hurt you. Not even the sea."

CHAPTER 4—RETURN TO PURGATORY
September 1966

On a crisp September morning, after five weeks at home between school terms, Lily boarded a plane bound for the city near her college. At the top of the portable steps leading up to the doorway, she carefully attached a cheerful expression to her face, turned, and waved good-bye to her parents standing on the tarmac.

As she entered the plane, the pilot greeted her, barely glancing at her ticket. "Hello, Lily, I wondered if we would be taking you back to college."

"Hi, Captain. I wouldn't miss flying with you. Besides," she said with a grin, "Student Standby tickets make flying cheaper than driving 400 miles. How's the weather ahead?"

"We're likely to hit some turbulence. But don't worry. This baby will handle anything Mother Nature can throw at her," he said, patting the side of the plane. "And I could land her in a field on one engine if I had to."

"Yeah, I know. Like you did in World War II. Totally safe. That's why I like flying with you." Lily laughed and, entering the cabin, spoke to the petite stewardess in a dark blue uniform who was tidying up the seats. "Hi, Nancy. I thought we were losing you to the Chicago route."

"No, I'd miss the smiling faces of all you college kids. Besides," she added with a conspiratorial wink, "Captain couldn't manage this plane without me—but don't tell him that." Lily glanced around for a seat. "Your favorite seat by the window in front of the right wing is open. I saved it when I saw you crossing the tarmac."

"Thanks, Nancy. You're a gem." Lily dropped her powder blue suitcase on the aisle seat and slid into her place next to the window. As soon as the stewardess moved away to talk to other passengers, Lily let the smile slip from her face. From her carry-on bag, she pulled out her journal and a pen and began to write.

"Dear Jesus, I don't want to go back to school, and I don't understand why. I love learning. I like our students and Profs. The college honors You. So why? I don't like the dirty dormitories and the fatty food. I'm tired of chapel three times a week and twice on Sunday. But that's not the reason."

The dual engines of the converted WWII bomber roared into action. The plane lurched as it started down the runway. Lily's stomach contorted threateningly. *Stop that, stomach,* she ordered silently. *You're only acting up because I'm going somewhere I don't want to go. So hush. I love flying and I want to enjoy this trip.*

Lily tapped her Lindy pen against her lips thoughtfully and stared out the window as the scenery moved faster and faster. Suddenly the plane bounced; then whoosh, they were in the air. Lily laid her journal on the empty seat beside her and, for a few minutes, forgot her problems. She loved the exhilaration of takeoff, of mounting toward the clouds, of looking down on the world. She leaned back in her seat and breathed deeply, simply enjoying the sensation of flight.

As the plane leveled out and the "Fasten Seat Belt" sign was turned off, she started writing again. "Up here, I'm free --like an eagle. But at home, I've never been free. As a kid, I had to beg permission to ride my bike when other kids yelled, 'Bye Mom, I'm going to town,' and pedaled away. In high school, I was an excellent driver, but my parents were afraid to let me have the car for school activities. They worried that 'Those boys that hang around the parking lot might bother you.' Even this summer after being away from home for two years, I couldn't go anywhere without them. Always the stifling and irrational protection.

"The college is almost as bad—isolating us and

expecting unquestioning agreement with whatever they tell us. I've learned to ignore a lot of the rules; it's the subtle insults to independence that infuriate me.

'As it was in the beginning,
Is now and ever shall be.
Dependency without end.
Amen. Amen.'

"It's a wonder I haven't been expelled for a bad attitude. I have already criticized the school more than some of my friends who were shipped out. " Lily continued writing.

Twenty minutes later, a shadow crossed Lily's journal. She looked out the window at a mass of silvery cloud.

Wow, we are gaining altitude again, she thought. *We don't usually go this high. We're going right through the clouds. We're surrounded. Whee! I can't see anything; I can't tell what is up or down.* She wrote: "Being disoriented in the clouds is fascinating. But spatial disorientation on the ground is definitely not fun. So many days, I get nauseated just walking. Whenever I turn my head, I feel like I'm in a different world—a world in the back, a world in front, and one on each side. And my chemistry lab instructor expects me to hold an eyedropper over a test tube without touching the sides?"

The plane let out a groan and shivered. *I hope they overhauled this crate before it took off.* She wrote: "I guess I'm like this plane. I need a complete overhaul—perceptual, conceptual, and linguistic. Especially linguistic. Words are a perpetual problem. I get accused of lying simply because a word means something different to me. Sometimes words lose their meaning altogether. Sometimes I embarrass myself because I hear words that aren't there. Yesterday in the grocery store parking lot I thought a man said, 'Ha! So they call you fatso, do they?' I yelled out at him. He turned around and said, 'Miss, I'm sorry, but I didn't say anything.' I turned red and crawled into my car.

" Even worse, I can't tell if my words and emotions

fit the situation. Last summer, a girlfriend was moaning that her roommate just broke up with a steady boyfriend. I laughed and said, 'She shouldn't have loved in the first place.' My friend was horrified but I didn't know what I had said wrong. Once a senior guy whom I respect was talking about the famine in China. I quipped, 'What do I care about those people 10,000 miles away?' But I do care. I care a lot about people who are hurting or hungry."

The plane banked sharply, throwing Lily off balance, knocking her journal off her lap. She scrambled around on the floor to pick it up, fighting the whirring in her head, as the dreaded psychotic pathology began to seep through her mind. The warning light came on at the front of the cabin—warning her to fasten her seatbelt, warning her that worse was to come. She held her notebook tightly, writing fast to get her whirling thoughts onto paper before they could overwhelm her.

"Why do I do these things? Jesus, it's not me. Something takes control. I'm so afraid I will really hurt someone. You've got to protect me. I can't–" Without warning the plane hit an air pocket and dropped abruptly. Lily's head snapped backwards.

As the plane steadied, she scribbled, "My head is roaring. I don't want to go back to school! I don't want them to see. The authorities and spies for the administration—they'll spot my difference. I can't hide. Ow, my head. I can't see. I'm losing everything. God, get me through the rest of the trip to school. I–"

Lily found herself sitting in the city airport. How had she gotten there? She had blacked out long before the landing. Had Nancy helped her? Had she embarrassed herself? She would never know. Now she must find a ride the seventeen miles through the country to her college. From the public booth in the waiting area, Lily phoned the front desk of her college dorm. The desk was staffed by volunteers and had the only phones in the building. Lily made three calls.

No answers. On her fourth call, a girl responded,

"Hello, Glasser Dorm."

"Please help me get to school. I'm at the airport," Lily pleaded.

"Sorry, no one here with a car." Click.

Exhausted, Lily leaned heavily against the side of the phone booth. What could she do? Time was running out. Any moment, she was likely to black out again. "Oh, God, help me."

"Hi there," a voice behind her called. Lily turned to meet a dorm mate whom she knew only casually. "Are you stuck here too?"

"Yes," Lily mumbled. "No one at the dorm with a car. Or the girl who answered the phone just didn't want to bother checking."

"Hey, you look sick." The girl suggested, "Why don't we find out how much that cabbie would charge to take us to school?"

Apparently the cabbie needed the business. He agreed to take the girls the seventeen miles for ten dollars each. Though the sum seemed a fortune to Lily, who often spent no more than that in a month, it was the only transportation. A half hour later Lily stood in front of the colonial columns of the red brick dormitory, profoundly thankful that God had intervened where her own faculties had failed.

Six days later Lily reported on her vacation to Professor Filbert. She explained that she had become better friends with her father and had lost the old terror of him, terror rooted in many spankings and threats in childhood that she had not understood. When she mentioned the ever-present hallucinations and spatial distortions, the professor asked, "You wrote me that you had a physical exam at your family doctor's. What were the results?"

"The usual. IAYH—it's all in your head. Prof, I know something is physically wrong. I'm nauseated. I can't sleep. Every day at 10:00 a.m. and 4:00 p.m. I have trouble breathing and staying conscious; it doesn't matter if I'm in class or playing tennis. Prof, I'm scared I will do all this psychological work and still be sick. I can't take that. I just can't!" Lily's voice rose to a high wail.

Professor Filbert leaned forward, speaking sharply. "Lily, listen! Lily! It's not an either-or proposition. You're thinking in terms of black and white again. The illness is emotional, spiritual, and physical. Our job—yours and mine—is to deal with the emotional and spiritual now. If the medical doesn't clear up, then you could go for a complete physical later."

"No, I can't. Every time I try to get help from doctors, they do a couple of tests and say, 'It's all in your head.' Then they ignore me. I know it's in my head but not necessarily psychological."

Suddenly Lily's face twisted in agony; she grabbed her temples. "My head. The noises in my head. Prof, I can't stand it. Make them go away."

Just as abruptly the girl straightened into an almost military posture and drew a deep breath. Her voice grew quiet and controlled. "No, I will not allow that to continue. I stopped it."

For the rest of the hour, therapist and client discussed school relationships and vocational plans with a calm objectivity that should have alerted the psychologist. What he never suspected was that Lily, unable to endure the threat of the conversation and unwilling to let herself explode, had entered her fantasy system. The professor had finished the session talking to Lily's alter ego, Shawn.

Lily lived the next three days thinking of herself as Shawn, queen of a mysterious jungle island. Though, previously, Shawn had intruded into the space/matter world for only a few minutes at a time, now that alter ego dominated Lily's daily existence, insulating her from her own emotions. Insisting against all reason that she was still in control, Lily regarded Shawn's entrance into college life as her salvation. She wrote in her journal, "Thank You, Heavenly Father, for this escape. I am more relaxed, more controlled than I have been in months. I thank You that I have learned to switch worlds voluntarily. Perhaps with this safety valve I can function more wisely until we remedy the basic illness."

That Friday night Lily and Rebecca attended the junior class play, *Peter Pan*. The college auditorium was packed with students. As the lights dimmed for the second act, Peter Pan and his gang of boys marched across the stage singing, "I'll never grow up." Always overly-responsive to music and drama, Lily felt herself capitulating to the allurement of fantasy, felt the arousal of her old, you-must-never-grow-up taboo. She sat on her hands to hide her clenched fists as she fought for what little she knew of reality. But as on stage Tinkerbelle led Wendy and the boys through Never-Never Land, Lily felt her sanity mask slipping, knew she was losing the battle, and knew her will was becoming useless against the inexorable forces propelling her completely into fantasy.

She nudged Rebecca gently. "I have to go back to the dorm. See you later." Rebecca nodded in acknowledgment, eyes still fixed on the performance.

Lily sprinted across the dimly lit campus and up to her third floor room, locking the door behind her. She did not want to be caught in a state of total "otherness." Lily pulled a large gold locket from her jewelry box. Pressing the beads on the lid of the locket rhythmically, she mumbled unintelligible sounds. She had not used this ritual as a means of entering the Island since she had been in college. Now her fight was desperate; she must master or be mastered. She must control her own fantasy system or it would control her.

With her thumb, Lily's flipped open the hidden clasp of the box-shaped locket. From inside, she withdrew a series of tiny colored-pencil sketches--an island with a single palm tree, a peculiar squiggle that could have been a man in flight with arms outstretched, a smaller sketch of the same shape, and an assortment of crude drawings of trees, animals, snakes, and people. Methodically she laid the slips of paper on the dresser and sat on the bed, staring at them. Then, eyes transfixed in the distance, face turned toward the mirror on the dresser, she intoned, "I am Shawn. I do not have to obey Earth commands. I do not have to grow up. I can go to the island and be the child queen. My brother will care for me, and I will rule. I go. Ah—ee—too—mah—sah." Garbled syllables streamed from the girl's lips.

Yet with some still rational part of her mind, Lily heard familiar footsteps outside the dorm room door, knew that a key turned in the lock, recognized Rebecca's deep voice. "Hey, Lily, what's going on. I got worried when you didn't come back to the play. Then I heard voices in here like some of the Oriental students. Is everything okay?" she panted, out of breath from running up three flights of stairs.

Lily did not answer but, with a swift movement of her left arm, swept paper and objects from the top of the dresser into a drawer, slamming it hard. With her right hand, she grabbed her hairbrush and stroked furiously at her chestnut curls.

"Say, when did you start paying so much attention to your hair?" Then Rebecca caught a glimpse of Lily's face in the mirror.

"Lily, Lily, answer me. Turn around here. Tell me what is happening."

The girl on the bed turned around. Instead of the soft youthful features of her friend, Rebecca faced the stony mask of a woman warring with the universe.

"Lily, what is happening?" From some corner of recollection, Becca pulled an idea. "Who are you?"

"I am Shawn. Lily is gone. But in your world, we are one." The voice, drained of emotional energy, spoke in a monotone, as though generated by a machine.

Rebecca shuddered. Lily had told her of the existence of a secret fantasy world but Rebecca had not expected to meet its occupant. Under the pressure of necessity, Rebecca took charge.

"Show me what you put in that drawer. Show me!"

The woman on the bed obediently pulled out the locket and chain and slips of scribbled-on paper.

"Tell me about them."

Shawn pointed to one at a time. "The locket holds the world. I am Shawn, queen, child, yet wise. This is my land, the Lone Palm Island off the coast of India. No one can see it except when I allow; otherwise it sinks into the sea. This is my house and my throne. This is my brother flying between worlds to escort me. This is me as a small child learning to fly. The snakes, the trees, and the tigers are for Kali, old god of the Island, before I came. The crosses on the figures mean that I banished them. Tonight they were flaring in rebellion. But I went back; I crushed them. They will not soon trouble me again. I am forever young and they cannot defeat me." Abruptly she dissolved into a childish helplessness and, through tears, Lily looked up bewildered. "Can they?"

Rebecca knelt down and fastened her arms around her friend, holding her securely in the position that served as the key to trust between them. "No, Lily. The tigers and snakes and trees cannot get you. Just relax. I'm here. I will take care of you."

Lily laid her head on Rebecca's shoulder and sobbed. Finally, when she seemed to have cried out all her confusion, she sat up. "I'm sorry, Becca. I'm sorry you saw me when I was just Shawn. I never meant for anyone to see me when I was completely in the other world."

"That's okay. Tell me more about the island. Who are you now?"

"I'm Shawn, but I'm enough Lily that I can live in America again. I'm not totally otherworldly, I mean."

"Are you two people?"

"I don't think so. Not like in a multiple personality, if that's what you mean. I don't usually have gaps in my memory, like multiples. And I'm always me, not someone else. I know that other people can't see and hear what I see and hear. I have always said that Shawn and the Island are my fantasy system, but that doesn't mean they are not real to me."

Rebecca moved across the room to sit on her own

bed. "I don't understand. Fantasy is reality. You are you. You are not you."

"I don't really know how to explain it all. You are the first person who has ever seen me when I couldn't control myself. I changed identities on Prof last therapy session, but I was still in the American frame of reference and he didn't notice. I haven't really been wholly Lily since then. The pressure of the play tonight was too great. I knew I was going to lose control, so I left. I didn't want you to follow me, but I guess I'm glad you did. If you hadn't stopped me, I might have gone in so deep I couldn't get back to your world."

"I'm glad I stopped you too. I wouldn't want you to go through this alone. Does Professor Filbert know this happens to you?"

"No, I told him I had another world but he didn't seem interested. And, until recently, Shawn never intruded so boldly into the time/space world."

"I want you to tell Prof on Tuesday, and if you don't, I will."

At the therapy hour on Tuesday, Lily obligingly reported to Professor Filbert. "There is something Becca said I should tell you. She saw me go into my fantasy world. She met Shawn."

"Who is Sean?"

"I am Shawn." Lily straightened into the military carriage, head too high, voice too well modulated. "I am queen of the Lone Palm Island, but I live in America and take back the best technology and philosophy to my people."

"Well, Lily, that is interesting. So you fantasize that you are a spy, and your name is Sean. Sounds like you have seen too much television. Why did you pick a boy's name?"

"I never called myself a spy, and my name is not a boy's name."

"I'm also interested that you picked an island, a body surrounded by water. That may have sexual significance."

"No, I don't think so. The whole matter is probably not important. Say, Prof, I enjoyed your sermon in chapel, but I can't see how to apply it practically. How do you love your neighbor as yourself? What do you do, and how do you make yourself feel?"

The diversion and challenge caught the psychologist off guard, and the Shawn self successfully maneuvered away from the delicate subject of the Island. She knew that the current line of misinterpretation could plummet her headlong into total rejection of the time/space world in an attempt to prove her own existence.

For the rest of the hour, as well as the next three weeks, Shawn, the alert intellect, reigned.

October 1966

By mid-October, Lily Farmer had fully regained her own identity and was pleased to discover a core of solidity in herself that did not give way under the rattlings of her worlds. At their next session, Professor Filbert sensed the new strength and acknowledged its appearance by sharing bits of personal information about the retreat he had led the previous weekend.

Lily reflected inwardly, *He is treating me as if nothing is wrong with me, as if I am not crazy. I like the compliment, but what price?*

However, the therapist soon refocused the conversation on Lily. "You seem to be feeling better, not so frightened, more relaxed. I notice in class that you are more involved with the other students. Your control system has improved."

"Yeah, it's pretty good for a schizophrenic," Lily jabbed, testing him.

"Did I say you were schizophrenic?" The psychologist cut away at the diagnosis he regretted giving. "I don't believe I did."

Cold chills shook Lily at the threat of losing her

right to be ill. Balancing the threat of illegitimacy against the possibility of being disrespectful, Lily insisted, "You said, 'You have a form of schizophrenia.' Are you retracting your words?"

Professor Filbert flinched. "Schizophrenia is a cluster of symptoms, not a single disease like polio."

"Your class presentation sounded distinctly like polio." Lily's lips tightened determinedly; she could not let this threat slip past without confrontation. " Prof, you needn't be afraid; I'm not. I live with it. Usually, psychologists describe the symptoms—the craziness, the weird behavior, the hallucinations and delusions. But in the class lecture, you kept going until you dug down to the bedrock, the split. How did you describe it?"

Cornered by his own words, his fingers drumming on the desk blotter, the professor quoted from his lecture, "Ah—umm. Schizophrenia is a split between thinking and reality, between feeling and reality, and between thinking and feeling."

Lily pronounced her indisputable verdict. "I fit. You know I do." To herself she noted *Shawn is my thinking/feeling split. I'm not sure about the other splits.*

The ever-present whirring in her brain spun itself into a roar. In a quick ploy to channel the conversation onto less treacherous ground, while at the same time gaining information, Lily queried, "Why do I have difficulty with the reasoning processes of algebra and chemistry, inductive reasoning, from details to generality?"

Either relieved or overtaken by another one of Lily's sudden switches, Professor Filbert drew a deep breath and launched into one of his comfortable lectures. "A generalization begins with many accurate perceptions. For example, how are an apple and a banana alike? Fruit, of course. A child starts to form this generalization through many experiences with apples and bananas. Then his mind relates the details of his perceptions into a picture of an apple and a banana. Finally the perceptions integrate, forming the generalization of fruit." Prof doodled pictures of the fruits on his note pad as he continued the explanation.

"The same mental processes of generalization are used to get from specific chemical experiments to general laws. The same processes are also used to get from specific social experience to an accurate picture of the real world. Because you have lived with this split a long time, you have difficulty going between the perception and generalization, and therefore difficulty with inductive reasoning."

"Prof, about those pictures you've been drawing. You're going to think I'm dumb. But that is how I learned that apples and bananas are fruit. In kindergarten, my coloring book showed apples, bananas, and grapes in a bowl and the caption read 'fruit.' I made a point of remembering the word. Otherwise I would have said that they are alike because you eat them."

The psychologist was intrigued. "What else have you learned that way?"

"Everything, I guess. Remember times I have repeated our conversations word for word when you were interrupted by a phone call and lost the train of thought? That's my recorder-memory. In grade school, casual friendships seemed beyond my grasp, partly because time and events forever fluctuated—now my friend played with me, now she had moved away, and I had lost what happened in between. To hide my time/space lostness, I memorized everything I heard or saw. When I was alone, I recalled and analyzed the memories. What do I do about it?"

"About what?"

"About the difficulty with generalizations. It's ruining my science work."

Again unbalanced by her abrupt change of subject, Professor Filbert did not realize that, instead of wanting an answer, Lily was retaliating for the pain of self-exposure. She knew that she was putting the psychologist in a difficult position, that there were no answers to her impossible 'what-do-I-do' questions.

Shifting papers randomly on his desktop, Professor Filbert groped, "As your emotions and thinking grow closer together, generalization should become easier."

"Terrific. Say, Prof, about chapel today. What is this that I keep hearing about Galatians 2:20—about being crucified with Christ? I've been dead, self-crucified. You tell me not to crucify myself. The preachers say, 'Live a crucified life.' How does that all fit together?"

Lily effectively protected herself against the professor's prying any further into her inner world. She did not want misunderstandings between them. And she was honestly perplexed about the concepts emphasized at this college. She rationalized, *Valuable information to ward off a valueless hurt.*

Professor Filbert obligingly explained. "In Galatians 2:20.the word *I* has three meanings— I the self-concept, as you think you are; I the identity, the essential you that cannot be destroyed; and I as God sees you. I (self-concept) am crucified with Christ; nevertheless I (the identity) live: yet not I (self-concept), but Christ living in me (seeing self as God sees me). Sanctification is the unifying of the three selves in God."

"Great. Three selves times two makes six selves. Which three shall we stick together?" Lily commented aloud, including her extra self, Shawn.

"What?" the psychologist asked sharply.

"Oh, never mind. I was just goofing around. Time is up. I better go. Thanks for sharing with me.'

Lily fled toward the door. Professor Filbert physically barricaded the doorway. "Relax. You will be all right." He locked his steel gray eyes into hers, penetrating through the mask and into her soul. "I will see you next week. If you need me, I will be on campus this weekend."

CHAPTER 5—ASSERTING INDEPENDENCE
October 29, 1966

Saturday morning after classes dismissed, Lily skipped from the basement classroom into the bright sunshine, glorying in the release of a weekend of freedom. Grinning from ear to ear, Rebecca intercepted her. "Let's have a picnic. Let's celebrate. You're getting well. And I just talked with Pastor David and he said I am more stable. The Lord is smiling on us. Let's go."

Swinging down the sidewalk toward the dorm, the two excited coeds had nothing serious, nothing abnormal, nothing more on their minds than the exhilaration of a free afternoon. Lily glanced toward the circle drive to check on the effects of the fall weather on the golden maple leaves, but instead of seeing the trees she spotted a white Chevrolet.

"Becca, Becca, is that my parents' car? What are they doing here? What's wrong?" Two harried parents approached the girls. "Maybe someone died," Lily speculated.

"Or is going to. See you later." Rebecca disappeared toward the dorm to avoid the Farmers who regarded her as a bad influence on their daughter.

Appearing very motherly in her soft blue suit, Mrs. Farmer greeted Lily. "Hello, daughter. Are you all right?" The tone was tense and questioning—as though Lily might not be.

"Fine, things are looking up. I have several new friends. I'm secretary for the service league. Most of my grades are A's. How are you?"

No answer, so Lily continued, "It's lunch time. Let's see what the cafeteria is serving. Or would you rather go downtown? What brings you so far from home anyway?"

"Lily, we have a motel room in the city. We want you to stay there with us tonight," Mrs. Farmer said.

Lily curled her lip in disbelief. "Why?"

In his early forties, tall, silver-haired Mr. Farmer stepped forward. "We are concerned about you and want to be with you for a while. In fact, we want you to come home with us."

Go home? Lily was bewildered. She was just adjusting to school. But Lily had never talked back or directly disobeyed her parents. Submissively, she packed an overnight bag and joined them in the car.

Later, trapped in the motel room in the city, seventeen miles from campus and friends, Lily felt panic rising, her thoughts tumbling one over the other. *Why have my parents come unexpectedly? Why did they want me to go home? What is happening to me? Or my parents? Am I truly crazy without realizing it? Did Prof offer to be on campus because he knew I am disintegrating? Or are my parents losing it? Dear Jesus, help me. Help me understand and act rationally.*

Clutching at the remnants of self-respect, Lily sorted through her parents' confusing messages. A letter from Professor Filbert had alarmed them. *Where is the letter?* Her mother had destroyed it, but according to Mrs. Farmer, it was Professor Filbert's latest progress report and had stated, "Lily has not improved during vacation." *Why? I feel stronger than I have in years. And is Prof actually writing reports without my knowledge?* In the letter he had suggested Lily have a complete physical since "she shows concern about her physical well-being and may be worried about cancer." *Cancer? That had never entered my mind.* The family doctor had informed the Farmers that Professor Filbert lacked the competency to treat serious disorders. *How can he say that without knowing Prof?* A local school counselor had told the Farmers that Lily should not be in school if she were "that sick" and that "time is a crucial factor." *How sick? And how could he know without meeting me?*

Lily pleaded silently, *save me, oh Lord, for the waters are come in unto my soul. I sink in the mire and there is no standing.* Never had Lily disputed her parents' claims on her, but this time their story did not make sense. Feeling a faint courage, Lily laid out her "why's" word by word.

Empowered by undefined fear, her mother countered, "If you don't go home and your father gets cancer again from worrying, it is your fault." Then her father interposed a fear for his wife's health if Lily continued to upset her.

Unable to fight the battle of wills alone, yet unwilling to surrender her independence, Lily blurted out, "I don't see any reason to quit school or to go home. But maybe I'm missing the point, and if I am, Prof Filbert will explain so that I understand. I want to go back to campus and talk to Prof." She choked back a flood of tears; above all else, she must not give ammunition to the charge of "emotional instability."

Tension, like static electricity, generated by the clash of determined personalities filled the hotel room until late afternoon when the Farmers gave in and drove Lily back to the college. Supported by friends throughout the campus, Lily searched frantically for her psychologist. At the moment that internal reeling seemed to spell capitulation to an unjust world, Lily spotted the familiar baby blue Oldsmobile and its driver, Professor Filbert. The psychologist caught his patient's distress signal and motioned that he would meet Lily at his office.

Informing her parents that Professor Filbert would talk with her, Lily hurried to her room and told her roommate what was going on. Flanked by Rebecca and another friend, Lily rushed to the professor's office. When she was safely seated inside with the psychologist, Lily tried to explain her parents' demands and their vague innuendoes and hints of impending doom. But the more she talked, the more confused she became. Her story made so little sense that she wondered if Prof would decide that she was crazy. For a few moments, the meaning of the words threatened to disappear into chaos. Then Lily saw the sparks of anger glinting in the psychologist's eyes, and those sparks lessened her feelings of intimidation.

Squelching the irritation in his voice with professional expertise, Professor Filbert said, "Lily, you're a rational adult, twenty years old. For my part, I apologize for corresponding with your mother against your wishes. My last note did say that you had made little progress over vacation—the vacation when you were at home and out of therapy. I did recommend a complete physical examination but indicated no urgency. As for this family doctor, how can he judge my competency when he has never met me? If you insist, I will speak with your mother, but I doubt we will come to any agreement. Your parents interrupted my class preparation period this morning. I expressed my opinion then. If this is an emergency, then go with them. If not, interrupting your semester is not logical. Lily, you are an intelligent, responsible adult. You must decide."

Lily's mind rose to the professor's challenge of "rational," "intelligent," and "responsible." What choice was there—living with persons, even her beloved parents, who treated her as a crazy child or continuing the support from a man who regarded her as a reasonable adult? For the first time in her life, Lily refused to obey her parents: she chose to respect herself. Lily Farmer chose to stay at college.

Wrapping herself tightly in her remaining dignity, Lily said good-bye to her parents. In a brief moment of privacy, she whispered to her father, "I'm all right. Don't worry." But he got into the car without any indication that he had heard her.

The car rolled away, and Lily felt that all the closeness she had gained over the summer rolled away with it. Rushing blindly into the dormitory main-floor lounge, she grabbed the waiting Rebecca. "I've lost them. I've lost my parents. I worked so hard to become strong, independent, and free for them to be proud of me. Now I've lost them. Why? Why?"

Rebecca pushed her down onto a sofa and let her sob. Finally Lily relaxed a bit. "I'm sorry I'm imposing on you, Becca. But I'm floundering. What do I do?"

"Let's go see Pastor David. He'll be in his study at the church on Saturday afternoon."

"But he is writing his sermon."

"He will forgive the interruption: this is an emergency. He can at least pray, and you know God gives Pastor David what he prays for."

Tenderly, the pastor shared the girls' hurt and then comforted them with God's promises. "Psalm 27 says, 'When my father and my mother forsake me, then the Lord will take me up.' Lily, through this break with your parents, perhaps you will learn to stand in God alone. Though you feel only hurt and desertion, ultimately God will be true to His word to work out all things for your good." The pastor prayed for emergency strength and new growth for both girls, for healing for Lily's parents and that, in all, Christ might be glorified.

Outside the pastor's study, Lily half smiled, trying to encourage herself. "With that kind of security, I can't fail."

Over the next two weeks, a series of letters aired the wounded feelings of both sides, but exposure widened the differences rather than healed them. To placate her parents, Lily agreed to spend her Christmas vacation having a physical examination at a nationally known clinic.

November 1966

After psychology class on Tuesday following the crisis, Professor Filbert called Lily into his office. "Lily, under the circumstances and the increased stress, do you think you are able to finish the semester?"

Lily grinned. "I made the decision. Yes, I will be able to endure. I have to be."

"Bless your sweet little heart. God loves you."

That evening sitting at her desk, facing the dingy yellow wall of her dorm room, Lily wrote in her journal: "I am thankful for Prof's comment today. He realizes the price of my decision and the difficulty of just existing with the increased pressure. He also understands that I had to stand up for my own independence and he respects me.

"Dear God, thank You for helping me toward independence. After years of obeying everyone, I need Your power to stand against authority for what I believe.

"A green olive tree in the house of the Lord I stand,
Rooted in God's garden soil,
Tossed by life's conflicting winds,
Seeking a way to lean."

On November 29, one month after the crisis, Lily wrote: "Therapy is doing its job. The time/space/matter world holds together—front with back, up with down, time without missing pleats. I walk normally, not like a tightrope walker balancing on a swinging wire. Eating, running, sleeping, and breathing come as naturally as if they had never withheld their services.

"I understand my love-hate ambivalence, why I automatically hate anything I love, how it pertains to my parents and dependency. I am closer to accepting my parents' inconsistencies; though, in spite of Prof's telling me to allow them their humanness and accept them as they are, I still want to force changes in them.

"At least, now my battles—authority, dating, lack of social graces, and a super-sensitive conscience—though intense, fit into college life. God, help me deal with these and make me whole and free."

CHAPTER 6—GUILT CONFRONTED; GUILT FORGIVEN
December 1966

Crisp white frost crackled under the feet of students hurrying from the evening church service to the dorms, heads filled with Christmas caroling, hot chocolate, and dorm parties. Two stray figures hung back, consulting in hushed tones.

"Was that you Pastor David used as an example in his sermon tonight?"

"I think so, Lily—me and partly you."

"But I haven't talked with Pastor David since October."

"Do you remember Wednesday two weeks ago when I had a counseling session with him? You had begun the morning feeling guilty because you had not washed the popcorn dishes the night before; you had added more guilt when I dragged you away from studying and forced you to play ping-pong with me; you capped it by picking on yourself at noon because you hadn't been able to persuade that boy to stay in college. I was fed up to my gills with your guilt, and when Pastor David asked how you were, I said, 'Guilty,' which I then had to explain."

"Oh, Becca, you shouldn't bother Pastor David with my problems."

"Your problems? Your guilt habitually turns into *my* problem." The girls reached the dorm steps. "Let's get a can of pop. I predict a long night ahead," Rebecca said.

Inside, Rebecca propelled Lily through the swinging doors to the vending machines. Though Lily cherished the Sunday night pop-and-rap sessions, she had responded to a recent missionary challenge by promising to deny herself all earthly pleasures.

"Becca, I can't spend the dime. I'm saving it for missions."

"Oh, for heaven's sake, those kids in India will never miss ten cents. You will. You're always sacrificing for someone else. Tonight you're going to treat yourself to pop or spend the night alone."

Reluctantly Lily stuck her dime in the machine, and then jerked away. "I just can't handle any more guilt, any more pain."

"Then I'll steal your dime and buy the pop for you." Rebecca punched the Pepsi button, grabbed the can, and forced it into Lily's hand. After Rebecca had purchased her own, the girls went to their room and settled in for a long talk with Lily sitting cross-legged on her bright madras bedspread and Rebecca assuming her therapist's pose at her desk. Rebecca started, "Tonight we shall resolve your guilt and authority hang-up. I'm sick of it; you ache from it; and I will not let you go home for Christmas vacation living in a murky world of self-abuse, especially with the stress of that medical exam coming up."

"All right, let's get this over." Lily opened her can of Pepsi, sipped, and set it on the desk beside her bed. "But if I fall apart under your dissection, you promise to glue me together."

"I will. Attention—what is the one and only authority you must obey at all times?"

"God," Lily asserted. "Anything He wants me to do that I am able to do."

"Do you practice that?"

"Yes, if I am able." Lily stared down at the worn tile floor.

"Does God Himself expect you to do what is impossible for you?"

"No, Jesus understands me."

"What is the source of real moral guilt?"

"Disobeying God." Catching the implication, Lily looked up from the floor, her mouth pursed in a whistle. "You mean—"

"Exactly! You are not and have not recently had any real moral guilt. The last time I remember was two weeks ago when you faked sickness to avoid a chapel speaker who would have upset you. You have asked forgiveness for that trick. The stock of guilt you hoard is a purely neurotic, conditioned response to your own humanness."

Restlessly, Lily strode over to the window, looked out at the shadowed snow, and then whirled around, spitting out, "What about all the hate churning inside me?"

"What do you do with that hate? Kill people? Or attack them? Or wish God would send them to hell?"

"No! No, I don't want to hurt anyone." Shaking with horror, Lily sat down at her desk. "I-I just pray not to have it and work with Prof to relieve the turmoil."

"Can you stop the hate voluntarily?"

"No, or I would. There is nothing more I can do."

"Then does God hold you guilty for not doing the impossible?"

"No, I guess not. But what about all those verses on hating as sin?"

"The legalists have you programmed!" In irritation, Rebecca slapped her desktop. "Call their use of Scripture proof-texting and ignore them? I don't know! What does Prof Filbert say?"

"Prof says not to worry about those verses right now and not to apply an isolated verse to myself unless the context and rationale for the verse really fit me."

"Lily, doesn't much of your hate stem from accepting everyone else as your authority, from trying to obey conflicting orders, insulting orders, from being used as a doormat?"

"Becca, I never conceived that I didn't have to do everything I was told until you nailed me that day in the drugstore." Lily's voice was trembling but she held her head up and looked her roommate in the eye. "Remember when we were eating at a booth at the back of the drugstore downtown? I was dog-tired; you told me to go look out the window to see if it was snowing. I went to the window at the front of the store. Then you laughed at me. The temperature was almost 50 degrees. I was hurt and embarrassed because you deliberately made a fool of me."

"But you got the message," Rebecca chuckled.

"Yes, I stopped obeying, bowing and scraping, apple polishing. I stopped bringing Mary's breakfast to her, doing Jenny's cleaning job, editing Linda's compositions, excusing Cindy's nasty temper, and working Charlene's math. And I lost my friends. I die daily under the guilt of my stubborn uncooperativeness. But at least I'm not a sidewalk." Lily determinedly stomped her foot down flat on the symbolic sidewalk.

"Okay, but the guilt itself is unreasonable," Rebecca said, taking a drink of her pop. "Your guilt about breaking unrealistic, compulsive standards was what prompted Pastor David's statement, 'Most things are neither moral nor immoral.' Lily, God only expects you to make a reasonable effort to live by His written rules."

Lily trembled. The volcano of hatred inside her spewed bits of fire that seared her skin and reddened her face, venting long-buried emotions. Lily shrilled, "No! God requires perfect obedience, perfect submission. I submitted and I went crazy because I can't be perfect. God is mean; God is cruel; let us thank Him for our gruel. God hates me; I hate Him; only Jesus loves; Amen. Amen. God hates—."

"Lily, stop that!" Rebecca ordered sharply. "Do you know what you are saying?"

Lily stared out the window and into the darkness. Trance-like, she dropped each word, "Jesus—loves me—but God—hates me—."

"Lily, Jesus is God. God the Father is exactly like Jesus. That god of *yours* is *my* devil."

Lily dropped her head and covered her face with her hands, tears trickling down between her fingers that shut out the light. "I'm sorry. God, I didn't know I felt like that. I don't want You to seem like a tyrant to me; I want to love You. I hurt You. I'm sorry. Help me," she pleaded, and then became motionless, unresponsive.

Lily was lost from the world of time and space, transfixed between the invisible borders of heaven and hell, waiting vacantly for her doom. She had insulted the Almighty: she expected to pay.

Standing vigil, Rebecca watched desperately for indications that Lily inhabited the stone-still body. At last Rebecca caught the flutter of eyelashes, then a twitch of the lips. Lily shook her head, parting the clouds separating her from the Earth world,

As Rebecca's worried face broke into clear view, Lily smiled slightly and said, "It is over. I am forgiven. Oh, Becca, God understood and accepted me. I lashed out from regions beyond my control and He did not hold me guilty. I know the feelings will be there for awhile, but now I also know the Father will not condemn me."

"Hurts and confusions deeply buried smell like hate when they are unearthed. That's what Pastor David told me. But God alone decides responsibility for guilt," Rebecca commented.

"And He is the only authority who can," Lily added.

"Praise God, and let's quit for tonight." After a brief preparation, the girls rolled into their beds. Rebecca muttered, "Lily, turn out the light."

"Turn it out yourself. The switch is on your wall."

Giggles dispelled the night's tension, and sleep crept in.

CHAPTER 7—A VOLCANO, A TUNNEL, AND AN ISLAND
February 1968

Lily Farmer stared at her comparative anatomy text open on the desk in her dormitory room. Comparative anatomy was her last difficult class, in the last semester of her senior year. In spite of the continuing tension with her parents, she had finished her junior year with an A average. Now, if she could only fight through comparative anatomy and maintain rationality for the remainder of this term, she would complete her double major in zoology and psychology and graduate with honors. She could get a job and be independent. But at the moment, hopelessness and explosive anger threatened to overwhelm her, to sever her tenuous hold on reality, as her mind rebelled against the loss of her greatest sources of warmth and security.

"I must not think about that," she lectured herself. "I have to concentrate. I have to study." With determination, she bent over her textbook, staring at the caption beneath a black-and-white photograph of a shark swimming. Clouds of gray mist floated between her eyes and the page, distorting the words. "I will read," Lily asserted aloud. Pointing to each word, she fought to catch meaning from the dancing black symbols. "The vertebral column of the shark...." The traitorous words danced faster and faster. Gray clouds swirled around her head.

Suddenly out of the grayness, the shark opened his mouth and bared his teeth menacingly. His tail fins swished; his body thrashed wildly. Through the mist swam the great shark, his gaping mouth closing upon the white hand holding the book.

"No! Stop it!" Lily screamed, slamming the book onto the gray tile floor. *Lily, control yourself. Don't give in.*

Stay rational, she ordered herself.

In an effort to quell the rising tempest, that unseen force that was in her but not of her, Lily seized her pen and scrawled furiously in her journal.

"Separated, barred, from the one person who understood and could control this thing in me. Why did they— my parents and the college—force Rebecca and me to live in separate dormitories, caging me in this tiny room with a sniveling wraith of a girl? Can't they see that without Becca I'm sliding backwards?

"Last spring with her support and control, I was almost normal. I was socially involved, dating, and making A's. Prof was so pleased that he recommended me for a responsible summer job.

"I had even survived that abominable medical clinic my parents forced me into. Talk about useless. Those doctors could not see what was right in front of their eyes." In an attempt to focus her anger, she thumbed through her journal until she found the pages from December a year ago. "Here is where I wrote about that torture session," she muttered.

Then aloud she read, "Hades is a synonym for ignorance. For the first two days at the famous inquisition clinic, I wore my dependable 'nothing wrong' mask, resenting the doctor's intrusion into my privacy, yet yearning to be understood. I filled out their forms and answered their questions politely and completely, but they would not answer mine. In the cavernous waiting rooms, I fled to the Island for protection, but the nurses engrossed in paper flipping never looked at me, never noticed when I could not talk or move, never noticed a body without a soul. By the third day, I felt myself sliding toward exposure of my whirling thoughts. Silently, I screamed for Shawn. She emerged, arrogantly open, demanding attention of the doctors in the Earth world. Bluntly, she announced her pain and distortion, but she was so controlled that her declaration was not believed. At the final interrogation by a psychiatrist, I volunteered—as Shawn—that I had an extra world that drew me into itself.

" 'Fantasy is all right as long as you are in control of it,' the psychiatrist replied, never suspecting that, as I spoke from the Island, I considered *him* the extra world. He continued, 'You are working through an adolescent personality reaction, nothing serious.'"

Lily slammed the journal onto the dorm room floor. *Nothing serious!* She screamed in her head. *Impending murder is nothing serious?*

Instead of anchoring Lily to reality, as she had hoped, the memories in her journal were overpowering her. Terrifying, vivid pictures flashed through her mind. She saw herself the previous October, standing in the middle of her dorm room, fighting against the other world's order to attack the new roommate forced on her by the college. Defying the monstrous voices in her head, she had willed herself to keep her hands behind her back and away from the thin wisp of a girl.

"Get out. Get out before I kill you," Lily had pleaded amidst tears and gasps. It was a warning, not a threat, but the naïve coed stood rooted to the spot like a terrified native witnessing the eruption of a sacred volcano.

Lily lunged at the girl, shoved her into the hall, and locked the door between them. Lily paced the floor, screaming, beating the walls, and hoping to dissipate the wild, objectless rage. Visions of murder and suicide flooded her mind. She tried to call out, "Jesus, help me," but the words were garbled and true prayer impossible. One hope! Get to Rebecca. Becca knew the keys of touch and voice to overpower the tempest.

Summoning every remnant of rationality available, Lily shouted, "Roommate, stay back! I'm coming out."

Lily fumbled into her coat, rolled up her bedding, bundled it under her arm, and started down the endless waving corridor, her limbs held with robot rigidity to prevent herself from striking out. With one shoulder sliding against the wall for balance, she passed the apartment of the dean of women. The door was ajar.

"M—m-misses-s Livegood, I have—to go spend—the night with Rebecca."

White-haired Mrs. Livegood gasped with shock. Girls sleeping in each other's rooms was unheard of. "Is something wrong?"

"Yes, I—sick."

"I'll call Professor Filbert."

"He's off campus. I tried."

"Then you will stay in the college clinic."

The thought of that ramshackle house with glass and open space and weak girls playing nurse terrified Lily.

"No!" she screamed. "Not safe. Afraid."

"When you are afraid, call on God," Mrs. Livegood placated. "He says perfect love casts out fear. You must not love if you are afraid."

"Go to henceforth!" Lily yelled. She fled clumsily out of the dormitory and across the campus, dragging the edge of her bedroll on the sidewalk. Mechanically she steered herself into Rebecca's private room.

"Becca, help me. Don't let me do it."

Rebecca had grabbed Lily's arm and had stared straight into her eyes, assuming control. Lily had fallen to the floor, sobbing.

Now, four months later, Lily laid her head over on her journal. "I was safe for the moment," she said to herself. "And I thought I would be safe with Prof Filbert the next day. I thought he would understand what I couldn't explain. But he didn't." Tears of genuine grief came to her eyes. "He didn't understand. He wanted to separate me from Rebecca, to limit the times and places we could be together. He said that she was not healthy for me. I tried to explain my fear of the invisible volcano of rage and that I needed someone who could control it. He said he would be there if I needed help, but he had not been there the night before, and maybe he would not be there the next time. I tried to tell him, but he didn't hear. He mentioned that he headed the Disciplinary Committee. That threat was the ultimate betrayal. I couldn't trust him anymore. I wanted to, but I couldn't."

Like a sick, scared child, Lily crawled onto her bed and curled up with her back against the dingy wall, knees drawn up under her chin. "I was alone. Prof was gone. Rebecca was too far away. I am still alone. As always," she whimpered.

Since the beginning of winter term in early January, Lily had waited to be accepted for therapy at the university medical center in the nearby city, but she had received no communication from the clinic. *There is no hope; no one cares,* she thought. Her mind slipped into utter darkness.

Mentally, Lily saw herself walking through a long, dark rubber tunnel that floated through outer space. Suddenly, at the open end of the tunnel, the light flamed brilliant red and an explosion ripped through her body. Lily leaped from her bed and hurled a bottle of ink toward the flame, smashing it against the yellow wall. She flung books, clothes, and a chair at the blinding red light. In a frantic call for help, Lily screamed, "No! No! No!"

Silence. Vacuity. The sound had placated the red light, and it dimmed. Still floating in the rubber tunnel in outer space, Lily was cold, lifeless, without feeling. Some still-functioning bit of mind caused her to write on a notebook page. "Get Rebecca. Stay out." She shoved the paper under the door into the hall. She curled into a ball in her bed, awaiting her doom, expecting that this time there would be no help. Without hope, yet her ears strained for footsteps in the hall.

She heard no footsteps, but the heavy oak door opened gently and Rebecca's large form dominated the swaying room. "Don't be afraid. I'm here. Let me put your coat on you. We're taking you to the university hospital." Lily leaned against Rebecca, letting her do whatever she wished.

In the hospital emergency room, sitting on the examining room table, Lily faced a stooped, gray-haired woman with a Dutch accent. "Why are you here?"

A dumb question, Lily thought. *How do I explain a*

volcano, a tunnel, and an island to a strange doctor? "I got violent," she said aloud.

"What did you do?"

"I don't really know. Threw things, I think." Vision and hearing became dull gray. The gray doctor looked to Lily like a troll in her childhood picture book.

After a few more questions, the doctor pronounced the verdict. "Nothing wrong with you. You just need a boyfriend and some sex."

A glass bottle of saline solution nearby caused Lily to wish her inner volcano would erupt so that she could crash the bottle over the troll's head. Picturing the liquid running over the gray doctor, she smiled.

"You think that is funny, no? You are all right. We are sending you home. We will see you in the outpatient clinic next Monday. The appointment was already scheduled, but you are a waste of time."

The doctor disappeared through the door. All light at the end of the tunnel died; cold, lifeless blackness reigned.

Lily stumbled slowly into the waiting room. "Becca? Becca?"

Finding her, Rebecca caught Lily's arm. "They won't help me," Lily murmured.

"I know. I heard. I'm mad. She's a witch. Lily, I have to get you out of this fog. Look at me! Look hard so that I can stop the fear and you can see."

Lily obeyed. Shapes and noises took form in the background. She heard, ""We don't have a way back to campus or a place to stay here in town. What do we do?"

By God's mercy, Rebecca located Lily's distant relative, Violet, who took the girls to her house and later drove them to the college campus. Lily didn't ask Mrs. Livegood. She simply got her bedroll and a few clothes and moved in with Rebecca.

"If I don't ask, Mrs. Livegood doesn't say no. If she doesn't get near me, I can't hurt her," Lily commented.

And Mrs. Livegood did not intrude.

The next weekend Lily spent trying to arrange rides from campus to therapy appointments and back. Lily hated asking anyone for favors. She was sure other students would not help her: few had cars, and fewer had permission to take them off campus during the week. In desperation, she went to the home of a college administrative secretary who had been kind to her. To her surprise, the secretary's neighbor worked at the university medical center and was willing to bring Lily back to campus twice weekly when he got off work. Then the secretary, who issued the off-campus work permits, talked a male student into taking Lily with him when he went to a job in the city at noon. Lily was humiliated but grateful.

Rebecca also would be entering therapy for her increasing depression with a psychiatrist at the county health department that could be reached by public bus. The girls arranged Rebecca's appointments for their day off so that Lily could ride with her. But Lily's appointments were set for times when Rebecca had classes.

"It figures. I comfort Becca after her torture sessions. But who do I have? No one."

Lily's regard of therapy as torture ended at her first session at the university medical school psychiatric clinic. Instead of the glowering doctors she had expected when she entered the office, Lily encountered two grinning third-year medical students in ordinary attire of white dress jackets and dark pants. Feeling an immediate connection, Lily quickly modified their names to Lew and Woolsey—Lew because he had the looks and liveliness of a popular comedian with a similar name, and Woolsey because his gentle brown eyes, curly brown hair, and substantial build reminded her of a big wooly brown sheep. Lew perched himself on top of the metal desk in the corner. Woolsey sat in the armchair opposite Lily's and stretched his long legs into the middle of the room.

The three chatted casually about the upcoming national election, and about college and medical school. Then Lew popped a question that startled Lily. "Hey, you seem like a nice girl. What are they doing at that school that's making you so angry?"

"Angry?"

"Yes, angry. What else would you call ripping apart your own room?"

"Oh, you know about that." *Bon voyage, friendship; here comes the lecture,* Lily thought, bracing herself.

"Gal, something is happening out there. What is it?"

To her own horror, Lily blurted, "I hate being in prison. I hate chapel, being nice, wearing my dresses all prim and proper, and living with liars. I hate DC's and dorm mothers and CDI's. I want to live."

"Oh!" Woolsey chuckled deeply. "Sounds like enough to be angry about, but would you explain?"

They accepted her. They thought she had a reason, a right to be angry. Lily poured out her frustration over the rigid rules, the regular room inspections, and chapel speakers who shouted, "Sacrifice," but drove away from campus in Cadillacs. She vented her hurt about Professor Filbert's threat to take her before the disciplinary committee (DC), about Christian duty informers (CDI's) always lurking to report the least violation, about promises of help that ended with the knowledge being used against students.

Lew grinned broadly. "Woolsey, I don't think she likes where she is living."

"Would you?" Woolsey parried.

"No, I think I'd give some people a punch in the mouth if they said those things to me."

The idea of Lew punching the dignified Professor Filbert in the mouth tickled Lily.

"Now, what did you say CDIs are?" Woolsey asked.

"Christian duty informers—legalistic kids who think it is their duty as Christians to tell on the rest of us."

"Oh," Lew quipped. "Well, go tell your CDI's to keep their seedy eyes and flapping tongues away from you."

When Lily finally stopped laughing, she asked, "Is

this your idea of therapy?"

Woolsey's dark eyes twinkled. "You feel better, don't you? Look, until you're out of that institution, our aim is to reduce the pressure so you can graduate. Then if you need intensive therapy, Dr. Willoughby will handle the matter."

"Who is Dr. Willoughby?"

"Our super-professor, one of the best psychiatrists in the country."

"Do you tell Dr. Willoughby about *me?*" Lily felt honored.

"Sure, every week. And Dr. Willoughby may observe a session through the two-way mirror to see how we're doing," Lew explained, pointing to a darkened window in the wall.

"Yeah, old Lew here has a mean streak. Dr. Willoughby has to keep an eye on him," Woolsey quipped.

After she stopped giggling, Lily said, "Excuse my seriousness, but the college says I must have a written statement from a doctor for me to stay in school. They're scared of me or something."

"You're joking?" Woolsey's mouth dropped open in disbelief.

"No."

Lew queried, "You planning to burn down the dorm or anything?"

Lily retorted, "No. If I were, I'd have done it when I felt hopeless. Now I'll take my aggressions out on you two. Just getting out of that prison three times a week is a relief. And since I'm moving into a private room this weekend, I won't have to worry about hurting a roommate. Also, my biology prof lets me work alone in the lab at night to avoid the pressure of having people close to me. He even gave me my lab test individually. He's as super as your Dr. Willoughby."

"Woolsey, shall we suddenly become full-fledged professionals?"

"Why not? They call us doctor." Dr. Woolsey found

a prescription pad and scrawled, "To Whom It May Concern: In our professional opinion, Lily Farmer is capable of remaining in college and should be allowed to complete the term." The two young men signed the note and handed it to Lily with a flourish. "We prescribe a B.A. degree to increase your self-confidence and your capability to deal with life."

Lily skipped out of the office as gleeful as a second grader who had been sentenced to staying after school for a month, then had the sentence suspended.

A half hour later, as Lily said good-bye to the kindly old gentleman who had agreed to drive her between the medical center and campus, Rebecca hurried up to her. "Let's have supper at the Country Kitchen downtown. I can't stand that noisy, smelly cafeteria another night," Rebecca suggested.

The two girls slipped away from campus, avoiding the cafeteria windows that looked out on their illegal exit. That evening set a precedent for all future evenings after therapy—supper in the village restaurant and sharing of the events of the therapy hour in an urgent attempt to shrink the pain of disclosure. Verbalizing therapy's content also took it away from the artificiality of the office and made it serviceable for the real world.

CHAPTER 8—DR. WILLOUGHBY
April 1968

Six weeks after the jubilant return to campus from the first session with Woolsey and Lew, Lily stepped onto campus with dejection of equal magnitude. Rebecca met her under the maple trees by the semi-circular drive where Lily's ride dropped her off. "Why are you so down in the mouth? You always fly after therapy," asked Rebecca.

"I won't be talking to Lew and Woolsey anymore; their term of psychiatric service has ended. I guess they told me that would happen, but I didn't understand. Woolsey introduced me to my new therapist, Dr. Falls, and left. Becca, the idiot shook my hand! Doesn't he know the electric voltage of a touch? He asked me dumb questions like, 'Aren't you exaggerating your problems to get attention?' The world began to go dark and I wanted to tell him to stop his chair; he was drifting away from me, riding the black waves up and down." Lily sat down on the concrete steps of the dormitory.

"I held my tongue in my teeth to keep from blurting out that I did not want an electronic clown who used therapy as a funhouse and me as his entertainment. I wanted to cry out for someone to turn off the power that voided the force of gravity, propelling me into space, but I gripped the chair bottom and held on. He would have enjoyed mocking me. Becca, the hour was intolerable! I can't survive with an automaton for a therapist and no warmth in the week." Lily had begun to sob hysterically.

"Now calm down." Rebecca patted Lily's shoulder reassuringly. "I believe you. We'll work out a plan before your Friday session. Woolsey and Lew told you before to call them if you needed them. You've come this far. You'll keep going. God wouldn't drop you now; neither will I."

On Friday, Lily shuffled stiffly into the Medical Center and rode up the elevator to the third floor psychiatric clinic. She seated herself in a wooden armchair in the far corner of the stark waiting room, so that she faced the door where her therapist should appear. *God help me. My world is reeling; my legs are sticks. I fear the "Falls," but more I fear my fear. I must express my pain, but I must be rational. Help me think and help me talk.*

"Miss Farmer," a high-pitched male voice called.

Frozen with fear, Lily could not stimulate her body into motion. "Miss Farmer, are you there?" Dr. Falls glared across the room, seeming not to recognize her.

With immense concentration, Lily managed, "Yes, just a minute."

"I'll be waiting in room three when you are ready."

Lily forced her eyes to see the waiting area, but it looked like a cartoon picture—flat, distant, and oscillating dangerously. Drawing her own aura around her, Lily entered the picture and plunged across the room and down the long narrow hall rolling like a boat on the sea. Vision refused to register the gold numbers above each door, so Lily entered the third open one. She grabbed the wildly weaving chair and fell into it.

Minutes later, Falls appeared in the doorway. "What are you doing in here? I said room three."

"I can't read right now," Lily stammered.

"Of course you can." Falls reached for her hand.

'Don't touch me," she warned.

Falls snatched at her upper arm, grazing it. The electricity of the touch broke through Lily's frozenness, and she came out fighting.

"You're dumb. You're stupid. You're trying to destroy me. I hate you."

The terrified girl rushed back through the hallway and into the open waiting room elevator. She jabbed the button for the first floor and the elevator obeyed. *Have to talk. Call Woolsey and Lew and tell them to call off the dog. Can't get any worse than staying in a room with Falls.*

Imploring her body to assist her, Lily found a pay-phone booth in the lobby and dialed the medical school number. She heard herself tell the operator this was an emergency call for Dr. Woolsey and Dr. Lew who were in class in pediatrics.

As the operator's page carried over the loud speaker, panic whipped through Lily. What if they didn't come? What next? Just as she was beginning to lose contact with the world, a voice said, "Hello. Hello. This is Edward Woolsey. Who is calling?"

Lily cried out in relief, "its Lily. Help me."

"Where are you? What happened?"

"In the hospital lobby. The new guy–Falls–he's stupid. I can't stand the power, his electricity, and my fire. Blow-up."

"Stay put. Don't move out of that phone booth. Lew and I will be right there. Will you stay put?"

"Yes, I'll freeze. Say something before you come close. I can't tell–" With an energy available only to the disturbed, Lily concentrated on becoming an ice statue, so cold that no volcanic heat could melt it.

Minutes later—"Lily, look around. I'm here—Dr. Woolsey. May I touch you?"

Lily nodded slightly. Dr. Woolsey grasped her firmly by both arms, turning her towards him, commanding more strength than the volcano and the ice. Lily leaned against him, relaxing inside. "I'm taking you back to the third floor. Dr. Lew is finding Dr. Willoughby to talk with you."

Lily stiffened again. "Don't let Falls close to me. I'm coming to and I'll hit him on purpose."

"I won't even let you see him. And I won't let you hurt anyone, including yourself."

Under Dr. Woolsey's firm guidance, Lily ventured back to the third floor. *Will they admit me to the hospital?* She wondered to herself. *I hope so. I'm tired.*

Safely deposited on a slate blue sofa in a comfortable office with Dr. Woolsey standing over her,

Lily's fear tapered into curiosity. She noted the two-way mirror in one wall and wondered if Dr. Willoughby was observing her. What would Dr. Willoughby be like? Would he wear the bland oatmeal face of the psychiatrists at the other clinic? Would--?

"Hello, Lily! I'm Dr. Willoughby," a crisp, New York voice reverberated from the doorway. Lily's vision popped into focus. A *woman*, bright red hair, fifty-ish yet ageless, stylish dress and heels, and smiling. Dr. Willoughby seated herself in a chair quite close to Lily and laid her clipboard on the desk. "I hear that you and my student aren't getting along. What is he doing that upsets you?"

No condemnation, no inference that she was guilty, Lily noted. She raised her head at the assumption that she had a reason to be upset. Lily opened her mouth to speak but felt that her first words made little sense. Whether they were words at all or just sounds, she was unsure.

She scrutinized Dr. Willoughby's face for the "she's crazy" expression or the more devastating counselor's mask. Instead she watched an amused smile play across the doctor's lips. The rest of the hour was a warm blur.

After a few minutes, Dr. Willoughby dismissed her "boys" to return to class, saying that Lily no longer felt explosive. Lily marveled that the doctor knew her feelings without being told. Lily rarely laughed, but she unintentionally giggled at Dr. Willoughby's well-placed slams toward persons who had disrupted Lily's life.

When Dr. Willoughby observed, "You're feeling much better, aren't you?" Lily had to admit she was.

"Have you read this book?" Dr. Willoughby asked, holding up a paperback with a picture of a girl among rose briars on the black cover.

"No, Rebecca wouldn't let me."

"Tell Rebecca that Dr. Willoughby, *your* psychiatrist, ordered you to read it. I think you will find a friend in its Debbie and feel less lonely."

"All right, I will." Then Lily caught her breath, eyes

widening. "How did you know I am lonely? I don't admit that even to myself."

"My dear, I have been in this business for many years. I know a lonely young lady when I see one. Also, I want you to ignore those preachers who condemn you. Your Bible says that God is love. Accept His love. I can understand and love you. If your God can't do as much as I, He isn't much of a God."

"What about Dr. Falls?"

"I'll see what I can do. I will at least talk to him and tell him not to touch you. Go back to campus and finish the term. After you graduate, we will find something better for you. Good-bye, Sweetie."

June-July 1968

A month after meeting Dr. Willoughby, Lily walked across the graduation stage, honor cords swinging around her neck, received her diploma for a B.A. degree, and turned her tassel. Back in her seat in the second row of the college auditorium, Lily let her mind drift from the words of the closing speaker. *This graduation is not all I hoped for,* she thought. *I'm not going to med school. But at least I will be working in the medical center and can sit in on some classes.*

Lily had found a job as a research assistant in a technologically advanced biochemistry lab, and, though she had never taken biochemistry, she assumed she could learn on the job as readily as in classes. She smiled inwardly as she remembered that working in this lab placed her only two floors away from the security of Dr. Willoughby and her medical student therapists.

Three days later, Lily and Rebecca packed all their belongings into the economy car that Lily's parents had sacrificed to give her and moved into an efficiency apartment near the medical center. Both girls were excited about their new freedom as independent adults. Although Lily had coached and prodded Rebecca so that she had completed her degree, Becca did not have a job and was not capable of fulltime employment. So the girls agreed that Rebecca would take charge of shopping, cooking, and cleaning and, until she was more stable, would stay half-days in intensive outpatient treatment at the state hospital while Lily was at work. Lily would be in charge of making the income, driving, and arranging evening activities. The friends were looking forward to long drives through the hills, picnics by the river, and lazy weekends at the park or zoo. They had no idea of the toll on physical resources extracted from the mentally ill by the normal world.

****

While the medical students were away on summer vacation, Dr. Willoughby invited Lily to come to her office for help whenever she felt upset. Lily went a few times, but, not yet able to accept the great lady's caring, she felt herself a nuisance.

One morning Lily awoke in her apartment to rumblings and shrill cries deep within her head and wondered how long she would be of this world. She opened her eyes to a flat, lifeless, cartoon room where each piece of furniture threatened to become animated. In spite of the anticipated danger, Lily stepped deliberately into the drawing and forced herself to get dressed and go to the lab.

Fumbling her way through the day's experiment, Lily cringed at the increasingly powerful roar from within. About 10:00, Lily felt the floor shaking under her feet, threatening to give way. The black laboratory tabletop rose toward her, blotting out the light of the world. From total blackness, she tried to scream, her mouth moving without sound. Her hand, which held a valuable tube of liquid, flew against the table, knocking the tube to the floor, spilling its contents across the gray tile. The crashing glass cut through the darkness allowing enough light in for Lily to see her destructiveness. In terror, she bolted from the lab and hid in a seldom-used restroom. Overwhelmed by fear and guilt, she curled into a ball in an orange chair and let herself sink into catatonic rigidity. A nurse, who happened into the restroom a half hour later, found Lily and somehow discerned her broken cry, "Dr. Willoughby." Before she could protest, Lily found herself seated on a velvet couch in the psychiatrist's office.

Dr. Willoughby was furious. "Young lady, did you realize you were getting upset?"

"Yes."

"Why didn't you come to my office?"

"I didn't want to bother you."

"When you are a bother to me, I will tell you. I can take care of myself."

There it was again—that unaccustomed acceptance. This woman said strange things.

Thereafter, Lily grew bolder, though from outward appearances she became sicker. As she felt more protected, her unconscious mind allowed larger and more virulent chunks of fear and anger to erupt into her conscious behavior. At the lab, Lily's work was increasingly incompetent. Her erratic measurements in the lab experiments gave the impression that Lily was lying about data; actually, she recorded whatever she could remember, which too often resulted in accurate first and last digits of a long number with a confusion of figures in between.

August 1968

In the blistering heat of August, the medical students returned to class. When Lily first met her new therapists, Earl Wilson and Tom Collier, conversation seemed inadequate to explain the chasm of internal darkness that separated Lily from Earth's bright summer. She labeled her wretchedness as exhaustion from responsibility, describing the tedium of an incomprehensible job and the constant vigil over Rebecca, now submerged in self-destructive despondency. Yet this description touched only the tip of the invisible mountain of fire that for ten years had been fueled by its own inexhaustible guilt and fear and now refused to remain covered by the mask of smiling stone.

That night, as the girls ate their supper of fresh green beans and potatoes at their small dining table, Lily verbally sketched the new therapists for Rebecca. Keeping her voice tightly controlled, guarding against her inner turmoil, she explained, "Earl is a favorite of Dr. Willoughby's, almost as perceptive as she is but much gentler. He is tall and the color of light oak wood. If my volcano blows, his kindness will shield him. Tom is short, muscular, and dark. He could handle an explosion."

Suddenly, like an eruption of volcanic lava, a mass of red burst across Lily's sight—red light swirling, churning, covering everything. Red flames everywhere. Through the whirling red, Lily stared, searching. Becca, she had to find Becca. She must be somewhere beyond the red, beyond the swirling holocaust. Straining, trying to see, Lily searched for the one person who could ground her to reality. The one person she must protect from the crackling flames. Where was Rebecca? There. Flames all around her! Her clothes on fire! Beyond her? The room, curtains blazing, blowing in the fire's wind. Everywhere—flames. Escape. No. She must warn Becca. Lily tried to call out, but only single words escaped from her throat. "Fire—clothes—curtains—run—escape."

Lily felt something soft and strong wrapping tightly around her, holding her in, keeping the flames away. With the gentle pressure, the fire went black. Then she was mentally gone, nowhere.

Rebecca had caught just enough of her friend's words to understand that she was consumed by psychotic terror and had wrapped a soft blanket around her protectively. Having been hospitalized herself, Rebecca knew the fear of freedom and open space to a mind running wild. For three years, she and Lily had leaned on each other like two walls of a tent, one holding up the other, alternately taking the lead, alternately providing protection for the other. Was their tent of mutual support collapsing, Rebecca wondered as she watched her friend staring in agony into nothingness. Were they losing all they had gained together, she asked herself as she saw Lily's eyes close and knew that her friend was dead to the time/matter world. For minutes--for an eternity--Rebecca listened to the ticking of the Baby Ben clock on the table, and watched and wondered and waited.

Finally, about thirty minutes after the episode began, Becca saw Lily's eyelids flutter, then open.

"Becca," Lily whispered, "You are still here."

"I'm here," sighed Rebecca with exhausted relief.

"I saw you burning."

"It was just a hallucination."

"It was more than a hallucination. It was a vision, a warning."

"It was a hallucination. And I'm tired. We're going to bed," Rebecca ordered, putting her arm around her friend's shoulders, nudging her to stand up.

After a minimum of preparation for sleep, the two girls pulled back the covers and sat on the edges of their twin beds, Bibles open from habit. Usually devotion time was warm and reassuring, but tonight it was different—cold, confusing, frightening.

"Becca, I don't know what to do. I'm afraid. It's like I was in nothingness and now the nothingness is in me."

"You are always telling me God knows what to do," Becca said a tinge of bitterness. "Ask Him."

"How? I can't feel Him. I can't feel anything, not even my legs."

At first, Rebecca was perplexed about what she should do: Lily always took the lead in spiritual things. Now Lily needed Becca to take the lead. Searching for something to help her friend, Rebecca flipped through her Bible, and then remembered what Pastor David had said. "Lily, Pastor David said when you can't pray, read. So we read." Becca turned to Psalms 69. "This is us. It's what I want to say. 'Save me, Oh, Lord, for the waters are come in unto my soul. I sink in the deep mire, where there is no standing…. I am weary of my crying…. mine eyes fail while I wait for my God.'"

They took turns reading familiar verses until Lily said, "This is the last verse. This is the way we ought to be. "Philippians 4. 'Be careful for nothing: but in everything by prayer and supplication with thanksgiving let your requests be made known unto God and the peace of God, which passeth all understanding, shall keep your hearts and minds through Christ Jesus.'" Abruptly Lily snapped off the bedside light and pulled her feet under the covers.

In the darkness, Rebecca heard a hoarse whisper. "God, You promised peace. Where is it?"

Before sunrise, Lily awoke, mind numb to the space/matter world, yet intently alert and striving. Quietly, without disturbing her roommate, she got out of bed, slipped into an orange work dress, and ate a bowl of cereal. Then absolutely certain that her evening's vision of fire held a warning, Lily continued to sit motionless at the table, head in her hands, letting her mind run through possible scenarios, hunting for an escape from her envisioned personal holocaust. *God, protect me; protect Rebecca,* she breathed, yearning for assurance that this day would not end in her own annihilation. Following subconscious directives, she reached for clean theme paper and began to write. In verse that flowed from regions of her mind beyond her control, she confessed her exhaustion and fear.

> *Infinite cold black tiredness,*
> *Crunching bone against muscle,*
> *Body whipped onward*
> *For lack of a backward*
> *Or resting hole.*
> *Mind cased in madness,*
> *World watching, powerless;*
> *Gone the resistance;*
> *Flames leap triumphant,*
> *Cheering, I burn.*

She added a note to Drs. Earl and Tom, placed it in an envelope, and addressed and sealed the envelope

Very early, just as the fiery sun topped the trees, Lily walked to the medical center and rode up the elevator. Guided by a small, rational part of her mind, Lily found her therapists' classroom and shoved the note under the door before the medical students were in the halls. She retreated to the lab, unlocked the door, and took refuge in a far corner until the staff arrived. Thinking out loud, she said, "A fool. I have to make a fool of myself to avoid destruction. I wish I could simply tell Earl and Tom I need to be hospitalized, but no one ever believes the straight truth. They think if you're sane enough to say you need rest and protection, you don't really need it."

Half regretting her own course, she prayed. "Oh, Jesus, I remember Becca's ward—the dirt, the seatless toilets, the lack of privacy, the weird-looking people, staff as weird as patients. But, Jesus, even that would be safer than the free world. Hospitals have volcano stoppers—medication, restraints, and here, Dr. Willoughby. I don't see her in outpatient, now that she's in charge of the ward, but maybe I could talk to her in the hospital. Jesus, can You make it be?"

She tucked her purse into a drawer at her workstation and said aloud to herself, "No, that's all wishful dreaming. Earl and Tom will probably ignore my note and leave me stuck in hell. Meanwhile, I can't afford to feel. Shawn, queen of bedrock, take away the feelings."

All sensation of touch, of emotion, and of caring, drained from Lily. Shawn's cunning mind performed the morning tasks until 11:00 a.m. when the lab secretary called over the intercom, "Telephone for Lily."

With dread, Lily picked up the receiver of the black wall phone near her workstation. "Hello, this is Lily."

"Lily, this is Dr. Collier. We got your note. Can you meet us in the student lounge at one o'clock?"

"Yes."

"Will you be all right until then?"

"Yes." She could think of no further reply and hung up the receiver.

At 1:00 p.m. in the medical student's lounge with Earl Wilson seated beside her, Lily wedged herself into the corner of the sectional sofa as though trying to merge with the beige upholstery.

Tom Collier leaned against a table in front of her, holding a sheaf of papers, some obviously medical center forms. "We got your note," he said in a tone that attempted professional flatness. "Do you still mean what you wrote?" Lily did not move. "Is there a possibility you were exaggerating, being poetic?"

She tried to answer, but found herself frozen in place. *Catatonic at the wrong time,* she thought. Silently, she watched as the two student therapists nodded to each other, and Tom slipped quickly out of the room.

Must talk to Earl. Mustn't block him out. "Mean the letter." Lily pushed out the words one at a time. "Can't go to apartment. Afraid. Can't fight anymore." Lily trembled silently; what had she just done? She scanned Earl's face for the "she's crazy" expression.

"Lily, would you like a vacation for a week?" Dr. Wilson asked gently. As she started to pull away from him, he moved closer, firmly taking her hands. "You're tired. You need to rest."

"Where?" *Vacation? Have I been so bad that he is sending me away? Better escape.* She started to stand, to run.

The doctor grasped her firmly by the shoulders. " You don't need to be afraid. You are going to Dr. Willoughby's ward."

"Oh." She let out a pained sigh and nodded.

Unsure what his patient meant, Dr. Wilson continued, "You will be safe. It is quiet there. You can let someone else take the responsibilities for a while."

Responsibility? Becca is my responsibility. No matter what it cost her, she had to ask. "Rebecca—will you tell her—get to state hospital? She'll kill herself alone."

Aware of Lily's determined caring, Earl reassured her, "I know Rebecca's social worker. I'll call him and he will do the rest."

Lily was silent for a few moments. "Okay, I can go." She stood, staring intently at Earl, searching through vast spaces for his reassuring strength. "I can. I can do it."

Earl took Lily's arm, steadying her, guiding her. "We'll walk over to the ward. It's just a little way. Dr. Collier has gone to talk to Dr. Willoughby."

CHAPTER 9—THE WARD
August—September 1968

  Shuffling between two heavy wooden swinging doors, Lily stared down a long hallway. Propelled by Earl's grip on her arm, she moved forward step by reluctant step. Before her loomed another set of doors. Panic choked her as she heard the strong bolt being unlocked. Her last chance. *Run. Turn back now or perhaps forever lose your freedom,* her mind shouted. *Run—to where? No recourse.* Lily stepped inside and knew the sickening rasp of the lock that has haunted mental patients for centuries. What she had voicelessly pleaded for was hers, and she wondered why she had wanted it.

  In minutes, Lily found herself sitting in a blue-green room decorated like a college dorm, but cleaner and more attractive than hers had been. Two couches with bolsters and blue and green plaid spreads converted into patient beds. The fragrance of fresh pine permeated the room. The private bathroom had a toilet with a seat and a door that locked. Lily's terror began to fade.

  "Hello, I'm Miss Thomas, your nurse today." A voice deep enough to be Earl's drifted from a small woman in street clothes standing beside her, checking Lily's purse. "Your name is Lily? Farmer? We're glad to have you with us on third floor. I hope you'll be able to relax and feel better soon. We have many activities and want you to join in. Feel free to come out and meet the other patients. I will take your billfold and keys to the nurses' station for safekeeping. You may get them when your doctor thinks you need them. Oh, there's the intercom. Excuse me. I'm being paged to the station."

  There was that acceptance again. Not crazy. Not condemned. Not suspected of hidden crimes. Earl had said "a vacation." Could this truly be a vacation?

From the wide halls Lily heard laughter and running feet. She stuck her head out the doorway, just in time to be narrowly missed by two teen-age girls gleefully chasing a boy down the hall. Where were the chains, the drab hospital robes, and the reigning specters in white doling out sedatives to hush patients' cries? Instead of the isolation and despondency she had expected to feel from reading about psychiatric hospitals, Lily felt her spirits soar. It was as though, with her hidden crime of weirdness now confessed, she had been offered an opportunity to live again.

Soon, teen-agers Bonnie and Margaret had dragged Lily into their lighthearted schemes. Their pal Randy would be leaving the ward the next day, going home against his wishes, and they were planning a party for him. Could they hide the cake and decorations in Lily's room where Randy would not find them, the two girls asked her in the twangy accent of the Appalachian foothills. And would she save her banana peel from supper for a game?

After supper, the fun began. "Come on," giggled stocky fifteen-year-old Bonnie, bouncing on her toes and bobbing her blonde head. "Let's play whiffle ball in the hall to get Randy's mind off going home."

Lily was in glory. Joining in the hilarity of her younger friends, she ran and chased, played tag and hide-and-seek, and forgot her age and illness. Putting one shoe on a banana peel and sliding along the well-waxed hall floor, Lily called, "Watch out, Bonnie. I'll catch you yet."

"Hot doggie, look at her skate," Bonnie cried. "She ain't bad for a damn Yankee."

"Damn Yankee, my foot!" Lily laughed, pulling the smaller Bonnie down to the floor. "I've got as much Southern blood in me as you do."

Margaret skidded on her banana peel and landed on top of them, her long dark hair falling over her heart-shaped face. "Then why don't you talk right? You talk like one of them city people from up north."

"Guess ya'll haf to teach her to talk after I'm gone," Randy chimed in. "Uh-oh, here comes Perky."

As the orderly approached, feigning irritation and shaking his finger at them, the three teens and Lily raced into her room, giggling and making catcalls at the white-uniformed man. From Lily's desk, they grabbed slices of chocolate cake that she had cut previously and set out on paper plates. Moments later three medical-student therapists trooped into the room with a carton of ice cream and demanded cake. The fun lasted well after normal bedtime, until the martial Miss Thomas marched everyone out of the room, including the young doctors.

Lily was alone after lights out. *This is a hospital? I'd call it a chance to make up for those adolescent years I missed by being good. Thank You, Jesus. Amen. Amen. Just snuff out the volcano again, again. If it erupts, I'll lose my friends.*

For the next week Lily reveled in the antics of her juvenile cohorts. The older ladies and their knitting groups that once would have bound her to their primness were relegated to the status of *insignificant*. Within the relaxed atmosphere of the ward, Lily found that her vision and coordination improved. Her body was free to play volleyball and badminton, constantly frustrated desires during her high school years. She became a much-wanted participant in all activities, a bit of a leader, outgoing and friendly to new patients. Only occasionally would fear and irrational anger propel her to the solitude of her room where she could suffer without losing pride.

On Thursday, she donned her freshly ironed lab coat for the first time in a week, preparing for a two-day trial at her job before returning to the normal world.

"Hey, Doctor, I got to talk to you," one of the new patients called to her as she passed through the ward doors.

Doctor? Lily looked at herself in the hall mirror. Wearing the white coat of the same cut as the permanent medical staff, her ID badge, a tailored dress and heels, her hair smooth and her makeup in place, she certainly could pass for a doctor. *What a paradox,* she thought. *When I was a kid, I acted like an old lady. Now I'm almost old enough to be a doctor, I want to act like a kid.*

At work, Lily survived the teasing about being let out of the monkey cage. But by noon, the laboratory world of glass and fire and uncertainty demanded its dues of fear. When she returned to the ward for lunch, the double doors were unlocked, since no current patients seemed likely to run away. Lily fairly flew through the doors, through the halls, and into her room. Curled into a ball on her couch, she waited the seemingly endless wait—for oblivion or help.

"Well, Lily, what are you trying to tell us this time?" Miss Thomas, the head nurse, inquired briskly as she seated herself on the edge of Lily's couch.

"Nothing. I'm just scared."

"You wanted my attention or you wouldn't have made such a grand entrance." Lily was irritated at Miss Thomas' perceptiveness; she always knew the unknowable. But that same power in the nurse created enough security for Lily to let words flow uncensored.

"I'm afraid to go back to work, but I have to. My week is up tomorrow, and I have to leave the ward. But I don't want to go back to fighting the outside world. It's too tough."

To Lily's humiliation, tears trickled from under her glasses. Crying before martial "Tommie" Thomas was a disgrace. In an attempt to discount this slippage, Lily rationalized, "Miss Thomas, I have learned so much this week; I do not want to stop learning." To Lily, learning was acceptable; feeling was not.

"Well, don't. Who said you would only stay a week?"

"Earl—uh, Dr. Wilson—and I agreed on a week before I came."

"I'll see what Dr. Willoughby says about that. I imagine she will speak with you in the morning during rounds. Go eat your lunch; it's getting cold. I'm confining you to the ward for the remainder of the day. That's what you want."

Miss Thomas was infuriating—always two steps ahead of Lily's own awareness of her feelings, always confronting her with them, always intervening when Lily thought she should be disciplining herself. "Tommie, the Storm Trooper," Lily had nicknamed the nurse. But when Miss Thomas was on duty, the ward seemed especially safe.

Friday morning when Dr. Willoughby and her entourage of nurses, interns, and medical students trooped down the hall after their morning conference, Lily left her door open so she could be seen and sat on her bed waiting. She wished she could run out and announce, "Dr. Willoughby, I have to talk to you." However, since living on the ward, Lily had learned that the other patients rarely knew the great psychiatrist and so she had become more reticent.

"Well, young lady, I hear you had a bad time at work yesterday. Want to tell me about it?" Dr. Willoughby's crisp, warm tones filled Lily's room.

"I'm sorry." Lily hung her head to avoid the expected condemnation. "I should have controlled myself."

"You're sorry? What are you sorry about? You were frightened and you ran to safety. That's a reasonable action." There, it was again, the acceptance, the assumption that she was acting reasonably. "Why were you frightened?"

"I was afraid I would do something dumb like–" Lily bit her lip.

"Like what?" demanded Dr. Willoughby in a tone that would not tolerate nonsense.

No escape. Lily had never directly related her fear of and enchantment with fire and her urge to throw glass just to listen to the crash. She was ashamed. The feelings were silly, dumb. She could not give a full description now; certainly not explain that since she had arrived on the ward she had experimented with burning matches against her skin. Yet under the imperative to answer the question, Lily blurted, "Dr. Willoughby—the fire, the glass, the anger. I'm afraid I can't control it. I'm sorry. I'm a disappointment to you."

"Sweetie, you're not a disappointment to me." Lily stared up at the redheaded psychiatrist in disbelief. "You're expecting the wrong things of yourself. Somewhere inside yourself is buried an enormous amount of anger; I call it a lake of rage. That's typical of young people with your background. Until we analyze the source and deal with the rage, you will continue to be afraid of yourself and the world."

"At the base of my volcano is a lake of rage," Lily echoed pointing to the finger painting of a volcano she had done in occupational therapy. "I must redecorate my volcano."

Dr. Willoughby would not be diverted. "Are you working through your background with Dr. Wilson?"

"Yes, I see him an hour each day. I'm beginning to understand why I hate everyone I love and especially why I hate authority."

"I think you had excellent reasons to be angry with *past* authorities, don't you?" Dr. Willoughby paused to emphasize the point. "I want you to stay another week."

"What about Rebecca?"

"Have you seen her since you came to the hospital?"

"No, I'm not sure I want to, but I know I have to face her eventually."

"Dr. Wilson communicated with her social worker recently and she is safe. I'll arrange for you to have visiting privileges and to be able to call Rebecca. Have a good weekend."

Odd, Lily mused, *how Dr. Willoughby protects me in just the right areas. I have had unlimited walking privileges, have worked, shopped, used the phone at the lab, but she knew I wasn't ready to see Rebecca. Even odder, after I've been with Dr. Willoughby, I respect myself. She has seen my sickness, yet treats me as if I make sense. A sensible sickness, I guess.*

The second week of Lily's hospital stay brought improved self-control and the ability to endure the lab for a full day without capitulating to the fear.

Lily gained pride in her easy relationship with the younger patients on the ward; as her adolescent giddiness faded, they had begun to look to her for adult leadership. Only at group therapy and ward conference did Lily feel her inferiority. She berated herself; *I should be one of the medical students in the group, not one of the patients.*

On Friday of the second week, Lily informed Drs. Earl and Tom that she was ready to enter the outside world again. However, they insisted that she stay for the big Labor Day cookout over the weekend, a festivity planned for all the staff and medical students, as well as patients.

"After all," Tom teased, "The patient-staff volleyball game wouldn't be much fun without you." Lily beamed.

Afterward Lily had to admit that the celebration packed in more fun and freedom than the total of her previous twenty-two Labor Days. She jotted in her journal:
> "I like me and I like life.
> I can see and I think I might
> Become the person I want to be,
> Swinging through the world so free."

CHAPTER 10—FORCED ENTRY
September 3–15, 1968

On Tuesday, after a day in the lab, Lily returned to housekeeping with Rebecca who was even more deeply depressed than before Lily had gone into the hospital. To Lily, Rebecca felt like a dead weight about her neck. Yet, believing herself responsible for the friend who had given her the first taste of self-knowledge, Lily considered no other course than to support both of them as long as her strength endured.

Two weeks of incessant exertion at working, cooking, cleaning, and driving left their mark, and soon Lily knew she was slipping from reality. Once again, rooms seemed to shrink into shallow, dimensionless pictures of primitive art. The gray mist which hung around her head restricted vision and hearing to distances within arm's reach. Often when the city sights and sounds assaulted her senses, Lily thought that inanimate objects were conspiring to attack her. She tried desperately to persuade herself that the phenomena represented what Professor Filbert had dubbed, "just symptoms."

As she walked home from the lab one day, a maple tree that hung over the sidewalk thrust its branches into her hair and yanked it hard, threatening in a voice that Lily heard plainly, "We things will destroy you yet." In self-defense she retorted, "Trees don't talk, and they don't attack people." But her statement lacked conviction.

Lily knew she had reached her breaking point. That night Lily sacrificed her cozy habit of praying in bed and knelt on the hard floor, balancing with her elbows pressed into the chenille bedspread. "Lord, please send me back to the hospital. It's my only hope. I don't have any money. Please take care of the cost and don't bill my parents.

They've paid more than they can afford already."

Since the acceleration of her inner distortions, Lily rarely heard God speak, but tonight she remained kneeling, listening. The pulsating, gyrating thoughts ceased and a peculiar peace rested on her. Quietly, softly—distinctly different from the unreal voices of trees or Island beings—came God's reassurance. "Ask and you will receive. I will provide." For the first night in two weeks, Lily slept peacefully.

The next day the methodical parts of Lily's mind systematically constructed a battle plan to force her readmission to the psychiatric ward. She would have preferred to summon the feelingless Shawn to live out the next few days, but she knew Shawn had to be banned. Realizing that psychiatrists do not accept a person's statements of her own craziness, Lily had determined to force her strangeness into open society, and the controlled Shawn would only complicate her plans.

During her lunch break from the lab, Lily hurried to the bulletin board in the third-floor employee lounge and checked the psychiatric weekend duty roster of students, residents and nurses. The coming Sunday was the day of Lily's choice; all the personnel working on the ward that day were friendly to her.

After work while Becca cooked supper, Lily sat at the kitchen table, writing out a plan for the disbursement of her belongings—what to store at her Aunt Violet's, what to discard, how to pack the necessary clothes into an acceptable form for bringing them onto the ward. The most troubling obstacle was Rebecca: she could not abandon her friend.

As the casserole of leftovers bubbled in the oven, Rebecca sat down opposite her. "Lily, I have something to tell you." Lily glanced up perfunctorily, then down at her list. "Lily, please look at me. This is serious." Lily put down her pen. In a strained voice, Rebecca said, "I'm going back to my grandmother's in the country. I can't stand it here anymore."

"What?" Lily exclaimed, startled.

"I'm going home where it is not so confusing. My social worker got my airplane ticket and gave it to me today. I leave Sunday. I wanted to tell you before, but I didn't want you to get upset. Please don't get upset."

Lily was not upset: she was relieved. "Oh, Becca, I didn't know how to tell you. I can't do this anymore either. I'm going back to the ward. But I didn't know what to do about--." Lily stopped.

"About me?" Becca actually grinned and pushed her straggly hair out of her eyes. "Well, this time I'm doing something about me. You've done enough."

Suddenly overwhelmed by a profound sense of loss, Lily snuffled, "It's over, Becca. All our dreams. Our plans. They are over. I did everything I could, but I couldn't make them happen." Lily covered her eyes with her palms and sobbed.

Tears flowed too from Rebecca's eyes, down her cheeks, and stained her pink blouse. Eventually, Lily's roommate got up and went to the wide west window. The last clouds of orange-gold glowed low in the darkening sky. Leaning her heavy frame against the pane, Rebecca mumbled, "So where is God?"

"What?" Lily sniffed.

"Where is God?" Becca repeated. "You did everything you could. I tried my best. When we give all we have to do right, He is supposed to help. Where is He?"

The question was asked earnestly and needed an answer. Reaching out in thought, searching beyond herself, Lily came and stood beside her friend. She opened the door and stepped out onto the porch, her gaze following the deepening darkness under the trees. "In the shadows," Lily answered quietly

"In the shadows? How?" Rebecca muttered.

"God is in the shadows." There were tears in her voice but she held it steady. "Remember the hymn we sang so often at Pastor David's church when there was trouble. It started, 'Once to every man and nation comes the moment to decide, in the strife of truth with falsehood for the good or evil side,' and it ended 'And behind the dim unknown, standeth God within the shadow keeping watch above His own.' Becca, God is out there, in the shadows, where we can't see Him. But He's there."

That night as Lily pulled the sheet over her head to block out the moving shapes of shade in the room, she whispered, "God in the shadows, what once must I decide?"

*****

On Sunday morning the girls attended the historic Episcopal Church that had been their place of worship for the summer. The ornate building and the formal mass provided an expiation of guilt and a solace not found in the churches of their upbringing. Lily felt a tinge of gentle sadness as she knelt before the ivory crucifix for the last time, chanting, "Lord, have mercy; Christ, have mercy; Lord, have mercy."

After choking down their last lunch in the apartment, the girls loaded boxes into Lily's car and drove to Violet's to ask if they might store their belongings in her basement. Although Violet was away for a few hours, her college-age daughter helped the girls carry their possessions to the storage area. In sparse words, Lily explained that she was taking Rebecca to the airport and then driving herself to the hospital. She had left in the apartment one huge box that would not fit in her little car and wondered if Violet would pick it up in the station wagon. Lily apologized outwardly for imposing upon the family's good will, but inwardly she did not spare the energy for proper guilt.

Violet's daughter recoiled in shock at the thought of Lily committing herself. She tried to persuade the girls to wait until her mother returned. Perhaps her mother could help Lily and thus avoid the need for such drastic action. As Violet's daughter talked on, Lily calculated the amount of internal power she had left to drive her exhausted senses—about three hours of sight and speech remaining—barely time enough to deposit Rebecca on the plane and drive herself to the medical center. *Dear God,* she prayed silently, *don't let me black out and cause an accident.* When Violet's daughter went upstairs for a moment, Lily scribbled a thank-you note, and the girls slipped out the door.

After Rebecca's plane was in the air, Lily compelled herself to remain conscious and rational until she stood before the swinging doors of the psychiatric ward, the gates to both safety and hell. A friendly young orderly guarded the first set of doors, giving clearance to the carefully monitored visitors.

" I must see the resident on duty," Lily told him flatly. That resident had always been friendly to Lily.

"You can't come up here and demand to see a doctor. You have to go through the emergency room."

Wrong resident on duty in the ER, Lily's mind cautioned her. "No, that's not safe," Lily stammered in panic. To herself, she commanded, *Can't do this rationally. Got to black out! What happens, happens. One, two, three—go.*

Lily's next clear realization was that of sitting on a blue-green bedspread with a white-coated resident's cold stethoscope against her chest. "You can stay tonight, Lily," the woman psychiatrist warned her. "But the department head will not like your being here. Dr. Willoughby will have to talk to him about your future when she comes back from her tour tomorrow evening."

"Department head, phooey," Lily mumbled. She had no respect for that man. She had seen him lie to a manic woman and then secretly slip away from her when the woman simply needed to be taken charge of, to be overpowered with words into security, to be ordered to sit down and shut up. Dr. Willoughby had stepped in, taking charge of the woman, and later had publicly criticized the department head's deceptiveness. Dr. Willoughby would protect Lily.

The resident on duty escorted Lily into one of the patient lounges and indicated she was to remain in the open areas while the doctor went to the desk and wrote orders for the nursing staff. *Uh-huh, I'm here to be observed by the nurses for flaws,* Lily reflected to herself. *Curl up and escape to the Island, but no explosion until Dr. Willoughby gets back, or you'll end up in the hall a discard. Only good little girls and boys live on this ward.* Lily curled her feet up on the orange couch and hid her face behind a magazine.

Almost immediately, Bonnie and Margaret raced up to her and then stopped, staring. *I must look as wild as I feel,* she thought. "Not safe. Not tonight," Lily whispered. With the characteristic consideration of psychiatric patients, they left without asking questions, and no one approached her that evening.

Eventually, over the top of the magazine, Lily observed Perky Perkitts, the aide, trudging through the lounge, carrying her suitcases in from her car and depositing them in her room. With a knowing wink at Lily, Perky enlisted the help of her favorite young nurse to check in her belongings. To Lily's amazement, when she returned to her room, she found that her red rubber ball and all her books including her Bible had cleared inspection. The nurse had even "forgotten" to check Lily's purse and collect her money and keys.

Someone around here trusts me. Since she trusts me, it's not fair to misuse my keys. Otherwise, I would unlock my window screen and go sit on the roof awhile tonight. This place is stuffy.

CHAPTER 11—THE ROCK TAKES CHARGE
September 16, 1968

At seven o'clock the next morning, Lily's door flew open.

"What do you think you're doing here?" demanded the familiar authoritative voice. Lily was terrified until she caught the twinkle in Dr. Willoughby's eye. "A patient on my ward in bed at seven o'clock in the morning? Tsk-tsk."

"I'm hiding," Lily quipped. "Are you going to kick me off the ward?"

"You certainly came in an unusual way, but you must need to be here to go to all that work. You should have simply told me."

Again—acceptance. Dr. Willoughby had seen through her scheme, yet assumed Lily had a valid reason for her actions. No condemnation, even though Lily had put Dr. Willoughby in an awkward position.

"You will have a new therapist, Dr. Robert Woodling. I think he can handle you. He likes a challenge." Dr. Willoughby glanced around the room, noticing that Lily had already arranged her belongings for a prolonged stay. "I see you are reading the book I gave you."

"Yes, and you are right. I do feel less alone after meeting its Debbie. She is so like me. She even has a volcano, though it is more spectacular than mine. But the book also helps me to understand myself."

"Good, you and Dr. Woodling may discuss the book in therapy." Dr. Willoughby pointed to Lily's rubber ball on the shelf. "Why the ball?"

"To take out my frustrations. You said to work out the adrenalin from my anger. At the apartment, I bounced it on the patio. But I have trouble finding a place to throw my little ball around here. I don't think the nurses would like the racket if I bounced it against my door."

"With a ten foot wide hall, you can't find a place to bounce a rubber ball?"

"The only solid wall where I wouldn't be in danger of hitting someone has pictures on it."

"Then ask Mr. Perkitts to move the pictures. They are not sacred."

Lily grinned. The only staff member she could possibly ask to do such an unorthodox thing was Perky Perkitts, and of course Dr. Willoughby would think of him.

"Dr. Willoughby, I didn't work Friday, and I don't know if I called in. I think I better go to the lab today."

"Do you think you should?"

"No, but I have to keep my job."

"Why? That job is part of the reason you are sick. But go on in today and see what happens. Dr. Woodling will stop by after staff conference this morning. Keep me informed through him."

Lily began a sort of frantic rush at turtle-speed. She washed and crawled into her work dress and lab coat. She downed the late breakfast Bonnie had smuggled to her from the dining room. While standing in front of the mirror and struggling to tame her rumpled brown curls, Lily wondered if she could adjust to her new therapist. She had met him once, and his vigorous manner had contrasted uncomfortably with Earl's gentleness.

"So, you like this ward or something," a deep, round voice addressed her from the open door. Lily jumped. "Sorry, I didn't mean to startle you. Remember me—Dr. Woodling? What's your schedule today?"

"I-I have to go to work."

"Then I'll see you at 12:30." Dr. Woodling had positioned himself close behind her. She could feel the strength of his oversized body in its brown tweed suit and that strength gave security, in much the same way as when Professor Filbert had held her eyes with his steel gray ones. "I hear you feel violent occasionally. I think we can take care of that." Backing out of the room, he said, "See you this afternoon."

Brown. A round, brown, rolling man. If a volcano hit him, he would roll up the slope and cap it with a brown stone, Lily reassured herself.

About midmorning in the laboratory, Lily was called into her boss's office. "Lily, I'm sorry you're having a difficult time," her supervisor began. "I believe you want to do your work well. I'm not sure what is happening with you. But I have to place the laboratory first. I think you know what I mean." Lily nodded. She had lost track of all her messes of the past month. "I'm going to have to ask you to resign. I think you might be able to do other work at the university, but not in a lab."

"What are you going to put on my record? Can you recommend me for another job? I have to work. I have to stay in town." Lily struggled to control the mounting hysteria.

"I will note on your personnel file that you are ill and that when your doctor gives you permission, you can do a paperwork job. Here is your check for this month."

Lily glanced at the figure on the check. "But the amount is for the whole month."

"Our budget can take it. You can use the money, can't you?"

"Sure," Lily replied in amazement. Then, wanting to show her gratitude, she said, "Do you want me to come in for the rest of the week? I could wash glassware or make coffee or something."

"No, you can leave the lab right now. Thank you for your efforts. Best wishes to you."

Lily clasped the check, murmured a quick thank-you, and fled. By the time she reached the ward, tears and sobs wracked her body; reason wavered under the herculean load. She snatched at the protection of Tommie the Storm Trooper. "Miss Thomas, please, I have to stay here. I can't leave the ward but I might have to. I don't have any money."

Miss Thomas firmly escorted Lily to the lounge.

"Sit down. What happened at work?"

Lily dropped heavily onto one of the pastel flowered couches. "I-I-I-was–" The word stuck in Lily's throat. Lily, the most reliable student in her high school, could not have been fired. "My boss doesn't need me in the lab anymore. I can't do the work well enough. Now without the job, I don't have any insurance and I can't pay the hospital bill. But I couldn't handle another job either. And please don't send me home like this. Don't do that to my parents—or me." Lily gasped for breath between sobs.

"Calm down. I will contact the social worker from vocational rehabilitation. I'm sure she can make financial arrangements for you to receive treatment. Sit out here in the lounge and relax." Miss Thomas strode off to attend to practical business.

Relax? She's crazy. To get treatment—what kind—at the state institution? No, under the gruffness, Tommie cares; she wouldn't do that to me. And Dr. Willoughby wouldn't reject me—would she?

Several patients, including the silver-haired lady who sat in the corner knitting, asked Lily why she was back from work so early. At first Lily burned with shame at exposing the loss of her job, but instead of the expected condemnation, she heard, "I'm sorry, dear, but you will find another job," or "Good, you'll be here all the time." There it was again—acceptance. Not acceptance of her weirdness that she herself accepted, but acceptance of her worthiness, her legitimacy, and her right to be.

Hearing Lily's voice, Bonnie bounced into the lounge, cigarette dangling from her mouth. "Whatcha doin' here? Those nurses ground you or sumpthun?"

"No, I-I was fired. I made too many mistakes."

"Yeah? That boss is dumb. You're too smart to fire. But that's okay. Now we got you. Come on, Margaret's in her room and wants to talk to you. She's got a problem."

"Let her tell her doctor."

"Well, heck no. She shore can't tell him."

Bonnie dragged Lily by the arm into Margaret's

room. Margaret did indeed have a problem, a severe crush on her medical student therapist. Unfortunately, the handsome young doctor-to-be had mistaken the girl's flirtation for adolescent silliness and had flirted back, compounding Margaret's romantic fantasies. Playing "Dear Abby" excused Lily from her own dilemma until lunch.

At 12:30 p.m., Dr. Robert Woodling appeared, as scheduled. He escorted the red-eyed Lily from the dining area to her room. "How was work?"

He can take it. Lily's subconscious mind registered the thought and turned off its monitoring functions. Raw, irrational emotion spewed out. "I got fired. I hate people. I hate myself. I want to get rid of the world. I want to withdraw."

"Why were you fired? Because you are living on this ward?"

"I can't stay on the ward. I don't have any money. I'm going to have to sit on a street corner or something."

Dr. Woodling insisted, "I asked you why you were fired."

"I can't talk to you. I can't trust you because I can't talk to you anymore because I don't have any money because I don't have a job. I have to leave this afternoon. Where are my car keys? Oh, I know where I hid them. Never mind. Tell everyone I hate saying good-bye." As Lily moved toward the door, Dr. Woodling grasped her quickly, firmly, by both shoulders.

"You sit down and listen." He shoved her down to the couch and locked his eyes into hers. "There will be some way to pay for your treatment here. You are going to talk to the social worker and you know it."

"She will say like everyone else, 'Her parents work. They can pay for it.' No, they're not paying and I'm leaving."

"Young lady, you aren't going anywhere. You are not even leaving this couch until you calm down. Lie down. Now sit up. Lie down. Sit up." At first, the former football player's strong grip on Lily's shoulders assured that she would comply; then she succumbed and exercised willingly. The sit-ups drained away the chemistry of anger. As Lily's body relaxed, Dr. Woodling allowed her to sit upright. "Do you see that I am not intimidated by you? Now, I'm not leaving this room until I see that you trust me. What has been happening at work recently? What was your job? Why did it upset you?"

Rendered defenseless by his strong-arm tactics, Lily recounted her incompetence as a lab assistant, her lack of training for the position, and her fear of the fire and glass and acid.

"It appears your boss did you a favor by firing you. No one can feel good about himself when he is failing at his job. And your lack of training predestined you to fail." Lily looked at him askance. Didn't he know that she was always expected to be able to succeed at anything? He was as strange as Dr. Willoughby. Noting her expression but not pausing to comment, Dr. Woodling continued to take charge. "As for your immediate future, I'm going to see you at least an hour every day. Since you have the protection of this ward, it's time to work through your stockpile of rage. We need to talk about your school, your religion, but especially your home. I will probe until I find out what I want to know, so you may as well decide to tell me in the first place."

"How come you weren't afraid to grab me? I hit people. No one touches me." This time Lily did not mean her non sequitur as a diversion. She was asking about who this man was, why his unusual approach, whether she could trust him.

"If I'm not afraid of you, you won't hit me. Right?"

Lily grinned.

"Anyway, you wanted me to stop you. You don't like that craziness any more than I do. From now on you tell me if you are feeling crazy and I will stop you."

Lily tingled with excitement. "You understand! You really do. Most people think that if you're crazy, you're crazy all the time. You know better. And you're right, I won't hit you. I—well—I trust you.

Lily couldn't believe her own ears. She had never admitted a secret so vital to self-defense so readily. Unconscious processes screamed, "This is idiocy" and dictated that she divert the doctor's attention from her expression of trust. Consciously, she thought, *All right. All the way out in the open. If he wants to destroy me, let him do it now.* "Dr. Willoughby said we might discuss the book she gave me to read. In it, Debbie feels like I do, except I have insight and more control. Maybe you could help me with my fantasy world, too. It scares me sometimes, but I don't think the Island would scare you."

"Yes, Dr. Willoughby did mention that book to me. I'll read a section before I come to our meetings, and we can discuss it. And I'm not afraid of your island either. But I still want to know about your early family life. You can't get around me that easily,"

Lily thought, *Foiled at a trick I didn't even have time to premeditate. This guy is like the Great Wall of China. No way around him.*

Aloud she said, "When do we get to work?"

"Tonight. At eight. See you then."

CHAPTER 12—FORBIDDEN LAND
September—October 1968

"Lily! Lily!" Dr. Woodling ordered, approaching the couch in her room where Lily was hunched, knees drawn up, back against the wall. "Get off that bed!"

No response.

Head on her knees, Lily heard Dr. Woodling's voice breaking into her Island world, but she refused to exert the effort to drag herself back into reality. If she was going to be able to trust Dr. Woodling with the unpredictable chaos inside her, she had to know that he could control her withdrawal as well as her violence.

Perceiving Lily's reluctance to strain against the imperious powers binding her to the land beyond time and space, Dr. Woodling sat down quietly next to her, signaling, "I'm with you."

"Listen to me, Lily. Trust me. I'm going to take hold of your arm, and when I do, you are going to join reality. Do you hear me?" Calmly and gently, Dr. Woodling fastened his muscular fingers around her forearm. "Now raise your head. Focus your eyes on my finger. Look at it. Look at my finger." With his free hand, the therapist lifted Lily's chin, then moved his finger slowly before her eyes. "Lily, time is valuable. You must clear your mind. We have a lot of work to do tonight."

In sudden fear of her growing trust in Dr. Woodling and in what she knew she would reveal under his pressure, Lily ducked her head back into her cocoon. She expected the man to leave in disgust.

"Lily, you're afraid. I recognize your sickness; I recognize its legitimacy. But you have to talk to me. I won't leave until you do." No response. "Look, Lily, Dr. Willoughby has already told me that you escape to a fantasy island. She has told me about your family, your college, even your religion. But she also told me that you are a fighter and that you have the stuff to beat this illness."

"Dr. Willoughby told you that?" Lily had been deflecting the therapist's words, but the challenge and trust in that last statement were irresistible.

"Yes. Dr. Willoughby has faith in your ability to solve your problems and to become what you want to be. Trust her faith in you."

Resigned, Lily stood up. "Let's get started." Inwardly she commented, *He works so hard. Mustn't disappoint the dear man.*

"I've reserved the staff conference room just outside the ward each night," Dr. Woodling explained. "Staying near the ward will give you more security than walking out to the clinic therapy rooms. Also more freedom to yell or whatever you need to do."

Resignedly, Lily followed Dr. Woodling out through the ward double doors, into the hall, and then into a comfortable brown and blue room with an oval conference table in the middle and a plush sectional sofa along two walls. Obeying her therapist's no-nonsense commands, Lily seated herself at the edge of the couch--tense, suspicious of her new surroundings.

After lowering himself onto the section at an angle to her, Dr. Woodling asked pointedly, "Where were you when I called you a few minutes ago?"

"On the Island."

"Tell me about your island. Who are you there?"

Lily was silent for a moment, listening to her inner warnings. "What do you care?" she retorted with uncharacteristic rudeness. "Anyway, it wouldn't make any sense to you. You will just try to destroy my country, or laugh and call it fantasy like the shrinks at the renowned house of terrors."

Dr. Woodling blinked at this abrupt shift in behavior, then, intrigued, sat back and observed. Casually he asked, "You mean the clinic where you had the physical exam?"

"Yes. Only Rebecca has understood about me. She knew my real identity and that this Lily everyone treats is just a sick façade." Lily's voice hardened with a haughty bitterness quite unlike her usual fearful tones.

"Try me," challenged Dr. Woodling. "I've proved I can handle your violence and your withdrawal. Give me a chance to know the real you."

Lily straightened, feet flat on the floor, head held too high. With an artificial smile, she said, "I am Shawnandoah, queen of the Lone Palm Island. I spend my time in America spying on your technology, your government, your educational and religious system. The best of it I transport to my own people, but I am careful not to carry in the deceit and hatred of your world."

Deep inside herself, Lily quaked. The voice of her sister on the Island cried, "Careful, you'll kill us." Her brother echoed, "Or he will laugh at you and kill you. Then you will have to infect him with your rottenness." Lily mentally retorted, *Hush, I'm your queen. You don't tell me what to do.*

And aloud she said, "I used to think I was a human like you, until my brother and sister found me and took me to the Island for the first time. There I learned why I stood out from other school children, why my American parents made no sense to me, and why teachers instinctively separated me from the others—sometimes for praise, but mostly to point out my difference.

"My forebears had come from another world where time and space, light and heat, were bridged by a single thought. The thought was father of the man, so to speak. My ancestors had ruled the Lone Palm Island on this planet for centuries of Earth-time and no time to speak of in their own. When I was born, my mother was spying in America. She died at the mishandling of human doctors, and a nurse secretly gave me to my American mother with no one the wiser.

"For ten years my big brother and sister searched

for me. When they found me, my big brother kidnapped me and took me to the Island. The elders realized that I was the prophesied child queen who would restore the Island's glory, now faded by internal wars and abuse. I was not an ordinary child. I was—"

A heavy fog floated before Lily's eyes; a rumbling punctuated with shrill whistles assaulted her head. "No, stop it!" she cried, grabbing her head with both hands. "I will not be quiet. I will say the truth. I-am-not-human."

The sounds of an ocean gale whipped around her ears. She drew up her legs under her gathered skirt and wrapped her arms around her shins to protect herself from the spray and fearful winds. Over the tumult she could faintly hear Dr. Woodling's voice, strong, soothing, yet without meaning. She tried to explain. "Gone, the meanings are gone. I told. I will pay the penalty."

For the next half hour, Lily strained her eyes and ears, catching bits of light and sound beyond the storm, searching for reassurance of Dr. Woodling's presence. Though his words were lost, she understood that the therapist was on her side, a rock in the storm, not laughing, not mocking, not destroying. She marveled that the gale did not affect him—but then he did not even know it was there. At moments, when she was able, she tried to answer his questions, hoping her words were intelligible, using the automatic function of her mind to give the same perfunctory answers given to other therapists.

As the punishment's fury abated, Lily ordered silently, *The Island is not allowed to have storms. I am the queen. I will control, won't I?* The storm cleared.

Lily announced aloud, "It is over. I paid the penalty, and I am still here." A slight smile of pride in her endurance escaped through the careful mask.

"You have fought well. Take a minute to appreciate what you have done." There was a pause; then he ordered, "Now I want you to lean back on the couch and close your eyes." When Lily obeyed, Dr. Woodling knew he had found the technique that would give him control and give

Lily the confidence to work through years of pain without succumbing. He continued, "When I take your arm, you will relax and begin to feel more like Lily. One, two, now." Firmly he grasped her forearm in the same way as at the first of the session. The tension in Lily's muscles let go. "Now look up. Look at my finger. That's good." He paused again, then said, "You feel more yourself than you have all day. We can have an ordinary conversation."

Lily actually smiled at him.

"You wanted to talk about the book Dr. Willoughby told you to read."

Lily nodded, still smiling.

"Is your island like the country of the girl in that book?"

"Only a little. But she was a fallen queen. I'm spoiled rotten, but I rule. Her country terrified her. The Island is a paradise." Pausing, Lily quickly consigned the storm to the American world. "The girl in the book was really herself all the time. My exterior is Lily, but inside I'm Shawn." She watched the air as another storm threatened. She was not yet ready to face her identity.

The doctor prompted, "Queens are usually catered to, and spoiled aren't they?"

"I was so spoiled, so putrefied that my mother had to wash and iron my clothes and fix my hair even when I was in high school and would rather have done it myself." A childish fearfulness slipped into Lily's voice. "She had to be sure that the rot didn't come through the doll showpiece. What confused me was that my father seemed to enjoy my rottenness. He would cuddle me and croon, 'You know, baby, you're spoiled rotten.' From what I heard grownups say, only children are always spoiled rotten. No wonder the world stinks."

Dr. Woodling realized that Lily equated the old saying about children being spoiled with a physical rottenness, with her physical body. "How do you feel about your body?"

Lily's eyes narrowed and with whispered intensity

she replied, "I hate it. It's rotten, no good, and won't do what I tell it to. It drops things, runs into things. It won't hear and see when it should. Then when I want quiet, it magnifies each sound. My face looks stony when I want to love, and it cries when I am angry. My hands won't obey my brain; they play their own tune on the piano, no matter how much I practice. When no one is looking, my hands and feet tease me by stretching off into the distance, then swelling and shrinking. My body gets real sores or makes up sicknesses so cleverly that even I can't always tell which ones are real. Then my father or doctors probe at it. They hardly ever know what is wrong, or they say it is a bacterial infection. But they see—I can tell. The infection is just the rottenness in me coming through to the surface. My father even admitted it a few times when he examined me. 'Nothing wrong, just the meanness coming out.'"

"Whew. Sounds like you have a good reason to be frustrated."

Lily was confounded by his acceptance.

"Anything else about your body?"

Lily hung her head in shame. "I'm sorry. I shouldn't have said those things. God gave me my body, and my Sunday school teacher said we should be grateful for everything God gives. And in tenth grade, a dream told me to be grateful."

Dr. Woodling frowned, perplexed. "A dream—told you?"

"I had been cursing my body. One night I dreamed my friends and I were on a farm. A tornado was sweeping toward us, and I sprinted across the barnyard to warn the other girls. My foot tripped me. I floated up into the air. I screamed a warning. Though I was right behind them, they didn't hear me. Then I looked back. My body was lying on the ground. The dream narrator said, 'Powerless, a soul without a body.' When I woke up, I knew I should be grateful. I'm sorry I hate this body."

"That's all right. But your description of your body and what I see on this medical chart are a little different.

You have been subject to frequent infections all your life. Infections are painful for anyone. It is possible that the infections and fever also affected the brain itself. Clumsiness and lack of coordination are frequently signs of brain damage."

Lily protested the rationalizing of her beliefs. "But nothing showed on the EEG and that clinic couldn't find anything."

"Some brain damage is hard to detect. And I doubt you told those doctors what you have told me. Right?"

"Right. You're special."

"Infections and brain dysfunction are very human problems, not those of a queen from another world. I would also suspect that during those examinations when you were sexually maturing, you felt violated and ashamed. Your feelings of shame are more evidence of your humanness. Use your education. Think back on your adolescent psychology course."

Against her will, Lily admitted that Dr. Woodling was right. *The rock hard truth must be faced when it sticks up through the dirt.* Aloud she said, "I'm tired."

"You should be. You have worked hard."

No comment about her laziness, Lily observed. This man did not mock persons who worked with their brains rather than with their hands.

"Lily, you have a good mind and a strong will. If you set that will to get well, no one can stop you."

There was no condemnation for her willfulness, she marveled.

"I want you to work with me every night. We will undercut this thing that holds you back from a full life. Do you think you will need medication to help you sleep?"

"Maybe something to cut the pain during the day." Lily wished for Mellaril. She had experimented with Rebecca's and found it steadying, but she dared not impose on the medical gods.

"I'm not sure Dr. Willoughby will agree, but I'll ask her. Take it easy on yourself for the rest of the evening."

For the remainder of the week, Lily slaved with her medical student therapist, dragging forth her secrets, her hopes, her shame—confidences given because she felt the man's own strength would stand against the rage within her and stand without condemnation. If she were to establish any basis for a future, she felt it must be in this ninety-day reprieve from the outer world, ninety days allotted by state rehabilitation funds. This was her first chance for safe exploration; it might be her last.

In her therapy sessions, Lily vacillated between open anger and fearful withdrawal. More than once Dr. Woodling held her firmly, restraining her thrashing, shielding her from her own turmoil. In her detached moments, Lily wondered how long it would be until her rottenness would rub off on this rock man. Once, in spite of Lily's attempts at control, the volcano puffed out bits of red-hot lava, but, to her surprise, the doctor who was pinning her arms against the couch wasn't even singed. The mild tranquilizer allotted by Dr. Willoughby merely nicked a tiny corner off the pain and was, in Lily's eyes, a mockery. Vigorous exercise did more to give Lily control by letting off emotional steam in short, physical puffs.

Lily resented the ward's demands for a pretense of sanity at all times and its insistence that patients live in an open world of space and fire or lose its favor. Testing Dr. Woodling's understanding, Lily commented, "Help with control is nice, but the girl in the book was really lucky. She could let the whole volcano blow and still have help." A quick search of Dr. Woodling's face told Lily that he could not comprehend total craziness as being better than partial, fake sanity.

Intent on her one expression at the end of that Saturday session, Lily locked herself in her bathroom and ripped a pack of matches from its cradle of tape under the sink. A purloined jar of ointment waited behind the toilet, ready to treat any burn that might blister and ooze, drawing the attention of the eagle-eyed ward nurses. Unlike her previous casual meetings of skin and fire, this burning was compelled by Lily's whole being as an escape from the time/space existence. Match upon lighted match against her stomach and thighs melted the stony mask, draining away the invisible pain, releasing Lily into calm nothingness.

CHAPTER 13—FIRE / RAIN
October 1968

Sunday morning, one week later, Lily received permission to attend the university Episcopal chapel near the hospital. Episcopal services of Lily's acquaintance had been formal, quiet, impersonal rituals which neither intruded nor condemned. The stylized liturgy had vaulted her prayers toward heaven, even when her own mind found itself incapable of original expression.

To Lily's dismay, the tiny student church was friendly, drawing her into itself, threatening to reveal her sickness. The homily spoke of involvement with our fellowman as Christ's representatives, spoke of joy and health and peace. Absent were the familiar intonations of repentance and confession punctuated by the plea so personal to Lily: "Lord, have mercy; Christ, have mercy; Lord, have mercy."

Even God denies me the chance to plead my guilt, she thought as she rushed out the back door at the conclusion of the Mass. Hysteria welled up within her as she hurried toward the medical center, and, with it, came the voices of the Island priests seeking control of Lily. The priests mocked, *all the world's a stage and queens must go on acting. Your mask must stay in place and your spy cloak on your back. No one believes the word of an actor.*

"Like fun they don't! I know my illegitimacy," Lily retorted. "You take up your quarrel with Shawn. She will send you where you belong."

The high priest laughed. *Shawn is fading into a LILY. She taught us her Jesus religion. Now let's see where her God is. Our war god will reign, and Shawn will be his first sacrifice.*

Lily recoiled, knowing the priest's statement was

true. Seldom now could she transform herself into Shawn in full glory and power. Never since she revealed the presence of the Island to Dr. Woodling had that country been calm and still and beautiful.

"I will save Shawn. I, Lily, will burn for my guilt. And it is not yet known what fire can do," she muttered. To her rapid, awkward walk, she timed a chant, "I will burn for my guilt. Fire takes pain; let it rain."

As she entered the ward, only her frantic eyes bore evidence of her agitation. Placid mask in place, she nonchalantly picked up a book of matches from the coffee table in the lounge and strolled to her bathroom, locking the door. She bared her arm. Lit a match. No feeling. No release. Touched her stomach. Match after match. The intensity of the hidden hysteria fused into a trance. The match seemed to be the tip of the volcano, placing her internal pain outside of her body.

Fire takes pain; let it rain. Bigger pain, bigger rain. She lit a twisted paper towel, held it, and stared. She slid to the floor in the corner behind the commode and lit another towel torch. Though she had no idea why, she was careful not to allow the flaming paper near her clothing. She watched the sparks fly upward, oblivious to all but the relief brought by the outer volcano that burned away her guilt and rage.

Vaguely, unaffected, she heard shouts and pounding, as though in the distance. "Open that door, Lily. Someone give me the key." Her bathroom door flew open, bursting in on her trance.

Mr. Perkitts, the orderly, grabbed her with one hand while stamping out the burning embers around her with his feet. Smoke had betrayed her. "What do you think you are doing? You could have burned yourself badly."

Fire-rain belongs outside, she wanted to say, but instead snorted, "I'm not a child. I know how to handle fire." Fiercely, with a temper that she had never seen from her favorite aide, Perky dragged her to the lounge near the nurses' station.

"Stay here." Shoving her onto a couch, he went in search of a nurse.

"Some protection," Lily grumbled, looking at the book of matches on the end table left there by a smoker. She slipped them into her blouse of her green shirtwaist. *I get some relief and then protection that is no protection. Be a nice little girl and don't upset anyone.* To all the rebels in both her worlds and maybe to God Himself, she announced aloud, "I burned for my guilt. I said I would. Lily burned; now leave Shawn alone."

A kindly voice inquired, "What did you say?" Looking up, Lily saw tall, thin Dr. Nunez watching her with concern.

"Nothing," she muttered. Dr. Nunez was her favorite resident. With all her heart she yearned to run in shame from the loving man. She wanted his respect and now she could never have it.

"An aide said you were burning yourself. Are you hurt?"

"No, I was burning paper when Perky barged in. It was nothing." She wanted to scream, *Love me. Stop me. Tie me. Don't make me stay free.* But restraints on that ward were unprofessional.

Dr. Nunez squatted on his heels and gazed into her face. "You ache. I'm sorry. I've watched you and I like you."

Piles of rules for proper therapeutic relationships fell about Lily's feet and she marveled that this slight man dared ignore their dictates. With her whole being, Lily searched Dr. Nunez' face; his caring was genuine.

He asked, "Did church upset you this morning?"

"No, the freedom did."

"I understand."

Because he could ignore the rules, Lily believed him and answered accordingly. "You're older than my father."

"You mean I can't like you because I'm older? Why not? Well, I wouldn't put you through having to talk to me.

But I will call Dr. Woodling to come over if you don't mind." He asked her permission as if she were normal.

Lily relaxed under the respect. "I'd appreciate that. What about the fire?"

"I'm confining you to the ward. I don't want you hurting yourself even accidentally. Promise me you won't burn anything more today. Come see me if the pain is too much. Promise?"

Lily, who could never say *no,* promised and was thus bound as if she had received the longed for restraints.

"You're an unusual young lady. I'll be here if you need me." The resident drifted away.

Lily returned to her room and tucked the newly acquired matches into the bolster on her bed. She sat at her desk with pencil and paper. Without her effort, words flowed from the pen.

>"The life of one who's almost dead
>From lack of food or being fed
>Is like a song so long unsung
>Or like a bell so long unrung.
>Both are dead or seeming so.
>Neither has a hope to grow,
>To do, to work, or yet to make
>The thing that first cracked the break."

Lily sought escape from the futility in her poem, mentally groping for the Island. "Shawn, take me. Shawn, I want to go to the Island," she whispered. Lily felt the flying-pack strapped to her back, felt its jet propulsion lift her, saw the blue of the ocean slipping beneath her.

Shawn's feet touched the soft beach sand. Barefoot, she wriggled her toes in the hot grains. She was home. It was good. With a calm, regal demeanor, she strode into the center of her village toward her family's house. A girl about four years old saw her and bolted away in fright. Shawn called out that she loved children and not to fear, but the child had disappeared.

Women in the village square preparing the common meal glanced up and then away. Shawn noticed tension in the faces of the school children when she reached their learning circle under the banyan tree. The teacher, her best friend, mouthed, "Be careful." Shawn was perplexed. She greeted the class and, according to custom, began to elaborate on the lesson under discussion.

"Hey," interrupted one of the boys, "the priests said you are betraying our Island, bringing in a lot of foreign ideas."

"Yeah," joined another, "and telling the outside world about us."

"Students, silence!" she commanded. "Young people have a right to ask questions, but you must ask with respect and a sincere desire for truth. You boys are being impudent and defiant. As for what the high priest is telling you, he is trying to take over the government himself and is accusing me to upset you. Yes, I am telling you about the world and telling select people in the world about you. Mass communications are too much with us for the Island to be hidden any longer. If it is half as good as it has appeared, the Island will stand the test. If it is really a prison in disguise, it will fall."

Suddenly a group of warriors surrounded her menacingly. "You are a traitor. You are now our captive. You have told; you will lose your refuge. Seize her."

Fear and anguish followed Shawn as she ran fleetly to escape. She neared the ocean; the beach melted into gray fog, the fog into paper.

Lily was writing:
> "Oh gentle Death, wilt thou not thy love show
> Wilt not thy kindness grow
> Envelop me in thy arms
> And carry me to my only home."

"What are you writing?" Dr. Woodling's voice burst in on Lily's solitude.

The ensuing hour rocked with pain, fire, memories, and revelations. Finally Lily said, "Don't be afraid of the fire. Haven't you noticed that I always burn in the bathroom where there is nothing flammable? I wouldn't hurt other people's property."

"And yourself?"

"Only enough fire-pain to set a back fire against the volcano. This place just isn't strong enough for me."

Again missing Lily's hidden message, Dr. Woodling continued his questioning. "You have something else written there. May I see?"

"Only a comparison of my parts, Lily and Shawn. Nothing dramatic."

Dr. Woodling read the lists. "I think Dr. Willoughby would find this interesting. May I give it to her?"

"Certainly, but it's really trite. Don't bore her too long with it."

*****

Monday in her room after breakfast, Lily heard the usual commotion of staff and students returning from morning report. Dr. Willoughby was giving orders in her most authoritarian voice right outside Lily's closed door and she did not sound pleased. At report, the doctor would have learned about her patient's disturbed behavior yesterday. Lily trembled, wondering if that was the cause of her psychiatrist's stern anger. Shame burned through Lily's skin: she wanted to run and hide from facing Dr. Willoughby. Lily sought refuge in the only available place, her desk, supposedly lost in a book.

Abruptly the door was thrown opened and Dr. Willoughby's no-nonsense voice called, "Good morning, Lily. Please put down your book." Lily complied quickly and looked up at the psychiatrist standing directly in front of her on the other side of the desk. "I hear you had a difficult weekend."

Not *I hear you caused trouble,* Lily noticed. The lines of concern on Dr. Willoughby's face frightened Lily, but their honesty evoked trust.

"What did you hear? That I'm a fire nut? Dr. Willoughby, I didn't destroy anything and I won't," Lily said, in a tone that pleaded for understanding. "Remember that's why I fled here. It's just that I had to burn for my guilt."

"Fire frequently symbolizes two things, cleansing and sex."

"Cleansing, maybe. But I also need to pay for guilt. And I need a backfire to stop the volcano. This place isn't strong enough."

"Lily, you are so afraid of your own strength," Dr. Willoughby said in a tone that cut right through Lily. "You are human and have only a human-size anger. There will always be someone to stop you."

"Always?"

"Always, if only the police."

Lily yearned to cry out that the police come only after ruin is accomplished, and that, until Lily met Dr. Willoughby, no one had been strong enough to stand against the turmoil. But maybe Dr. Willoughby possessed power to decree a reversal of her whole life. She would see.

"Maybe," she replied. "My rule of the Island is being threatened. I asked Dr. Woodling to go there with me for a final battle. I must own my refuge."

"You must own yourself. When you possess all of your own thoughts and feelings, the island will be yours if you still want it." Then seating herself on the other desk chair, the psychiatrist said, " I read your analysis of Shawn and Lily. You first say that Shawn is a fantasy identity. Then you say you are really Shawn and Lily is a mask. But in reality, you have characteristics of both. And frankly, in some cases, I like Lily better." She smiled her smile of approbation.

"But Lily is sick. You can't like a sick person."

"Oh, I can't? Am I a doctor because I hate my patients? Then I'm in the wrong profession."

Lily laughed, and then said seriously, "But there's nothing in Lily to like."

"No? Lily cared about her college friend. Lily takes time with teenagers on this ward and listens to their heartthrobs. Lily makes sound suggestions at patient-staff meetings, overcoming a great deal of anxiety in the process. Well, I guess I just don't know what to respect—or your Lily is a different one than lives on this ward."

Lily beamed. Dr. Willoughby still liked her.

Then in the firm, no-nonsense-tolerated tone that pierced Lily's defenses, Dr. Willoughby continued, "But you must decide whether you are going to pursue reality and health or to retreat into your fantasies. You have the right to retreat, but do it all the way and take up residency at the state hospital. You will be well cared for there. If you decide for reality, you will have a long fight ahead, but I can assure you that reality is worth the fight. When you make up your mind, let me know."

"I'll tell you Friday."

CHAPTER 14 – THE DECISION
October 1968

Lily withdrew into a week of torment. She abandoned volleyball, occupational therapy, TV, and desserts. Of the patients, only Bonnie and Margaret dared approach her. Doctor's orders confined her to the ward, and she confined herself to her room. For hours, she poured over the Bible, her old journals, and psychology books previously checked out from the medical school library on her old staff card.

Did she have a chance to be "normal"? What *was* "normal"? Were the percentages of success worth the overwhelming effort required? Would she lose her Island and the other fantasies that drifted in as she needed them? Was reality anything but pain? At that question, she stopped abruptly. She was asked to live in reality. What *was* reality?

Thursday morning, she sat cross-legged on the tile floor of her room, painting out her hostilities with temperas. Margaret painted next to her.

"Margaret, is reality worth living in?"

Margaret, whose problems centered on an alcoholic home, grunted, "Uh-huh."

"Why?"

"Love, where you can find it."

Margaret painted, "I hate this place." Lily, determined to shatter her nice girl image painted, "I hate this darn ward." The girls giggled. They knew that it was the environment of forced decisions and self-honesty, not the physical ward that they hated. Gleefully, they hung the signs on the wall in direct view of the door.

Over her bed, Lily hung a painting of a pair of vicious eyes that had haunted her nightly after the lights were out. The conspirators laughed; they had had their say. They had violated the staff's false insistence that this ward was for nice people who were "sick." Lily crowned their announcement with a poster for the back of door. "I am nuts."

Freed by the externalization, Lily settled down at her desk, pen flying across paper. " What is Reality? Reality is that which has existence in itself and is not dependent on anything else. Reality. Love. God is love. Reality. God. God is Reality. God is the *only* completely independent being. All other reality emanates from Him. God, as the Creator of the real world, is Ultimate Reality."

She threw down her pen and, leaping from her chair, twirled around three times. "That's it! I've found my answer."

Then, invoking the tough-mindedness so contradictory to her childish emotions, Lily poured over Scripture references to the characteristics of God, substituting the word *reality* for other descriptive words. Would her idea stand the test?

God is Reality and in Him is no unreality. That was true. Lily had previously proved to herself that the more she lived in social and physical realness, the closer was her relationship to her beloved Jesus. *For God so desired to bring Reality into men's lives that He gave His only begotten Son that whosoever believeth in Him should not perish but have everlasting life.*

True, God wanted men to understand and side with Him in the spiritual wars that permeated the universe. *Know ye Reality and Reality shall set you free.*

"Oh, Jesus, it is true! Reality is You. Reality is not a giant waiting to snatch and devour me. Reality is my loving Jesus. You're the only Person I thoroughly trust. I've stayed alive and kept trying just for You. You are Reality, and I didn't even realize it. That means there must be order and reason and logic and good out there in that time/space/matter world because You created it."

Her enthusiasm subsided.

"Father God, maybe my theory is a trick of my mind. And there are still many unsettled questions. Pain, hate, hurt—where do they fit in? Hold me steady; let me think clearly; show me Your truth. I owe Dr. Willoughby an answer by tomorrow morning."

Lily listened intently, fixing her spiritual ears on a dimension beyond the reaches of hallucination. The answer came. "I am the Way, the Truth, and the Life. I love you. You and I can win."

Friday morning when Dr. Willoughby and her entourage swept through the hall, Lily stepped forward to gain attention. "Dr. Willoughby, may I speak with you?" She quaked lest the nurses tell her to go away, but Dr. Willoughby motioned her staff on to daily tasks and stepped into Lily's room.

"I've decided."

"Oh, and--?"

"I've decided to live in reality. Or at least to try to find reality. I know I'll pay for my decision, but I'm going to try."

Dr. Wilbur seated herself on Lily's desk chair, crossed her legs, and smiled at her patient. "I could see your decision already. You would not have stopped me if you intended to escape from life. You feel good about your decision, don't you?"

"Dr. Willoughby, what about the guilt and fear? Will I always have them?"

"No. When you find their source, they will fall away. That is why Dr. Woodling wants you to talk about your parents and your past."

Lily wanted to protest that she had told those stories repeatedly, with no change in her mental or emotional functioning. But that would be disrespectful. Instead, she dropped down on her bed, twisting her fingers nervously, and said, "I still believe there is a physical problem. I did my senior project on the biochemistry of schizophrenia, and there's good evidence for physical sources of this disease."

"My training is in psychoanalysis, and I still believe your disturbance is rooted in your past, especially in your home."

"My parents love me. They wrote, encouraging me to stay here and get help."

Dr. Willoughby's voice was warm but firm. "They love you as they understand love. But you need a love that says you have a right to be the person you are. Love that commends, but not constricts."

"And that's what you give me!" With this sudden insight, Lily fidgeted. "You're like a real—a—." Lily bit her tongue, afraid of offending the great lady's professionalism.

"A mother? I intend to be."

"You do? But—but my counseling books all say--."

"I don't abide by those books."

"You surely don't." They laughed—like cohorts in a scheme against the academic rules, Lily thought. She did not understand the psychoanalytic phenomenon of transference, but she felt its effects. "I wouldn't mind being female if I could be like you. But I was always taught a woman should be quiet, submissive, dependent, and incompetent. In churches I've been in you would be bad."

"Ignore those churches. You believe in Jesus. What did He say?"

Lily thought hard for a few moments. "In the Old Testament, God made Deborah judge of the whole nation of Israel. Two of Jesus' best friends were women and community figures. And Priscilla was a leader in the Early Church. So Jesus thought of women as competent and leaders."

"Well, then?"

"I get the point," Lily said, though she only partially understood.

That evening, Dr. Woodling and Lily confronted the old ghosts of guilt that constantly reinforced her feelings of contagion and rottenness.

As soon as they were seated in the therapy room,

Lily announced, "I have decided to live in reality. But as rotten as I am, that's too bad for reality. It's going to stink worse."

"Then let's get the stink out in the fresh air for purification. Name your guilts."

"The winter I was three, my father told me not to turn on the outside water faucet. I wanted to put water in a Vicks jar and watch it freeze. I turned on the faucet, but I couldn't shut it off all the way. It dripped. When my father came home, he asked who had turned on the faucet. I didn't answer. I became drip number one."

"In kindergarten, I was guilty of being too smart to play with the group and too dumb to write my name in pretty colors like another girl. In first grade I colored the wrong number of balls in my number book and no matter how many times I tried to erase, I always colored them back the same way. From then on, I had trouble in math and was guilty of carelessness. The A's on my report card were gifts to cover the bad smell.

"In second grade, I drew a picture of me building a snow house, when I was suppose to draw myself ice skating. I couldn't draw a picture of me doing that because I couldn't ice skate. I become guilty of willfulness. From then on I covered the underwear of willfulness with a dress of courtesy and was guilty of fawning and deceit. In sixth grade I almost killed my girlfriend in a pillow fight. Only *I* didn't do it. Something overpowered me; I blacked out and knocked her unconscious. That night and for many weeks I floated over my bed and then fell, hitting hard. I was guilty of both murder and the impossible. I wanted someone to tell me what was wrong with me. The Great Commandment says, 'Do unto others as you would have them do unto you'. So I told my cousin that her medicine was for epilepsy, a secret I had promised not to tell. I was guilty of dishonesty and untrustworthiness. I can keep the Commandments and be guilty of them at the same time. Pretty good, don't you think?"

Lily continued her recital without waiting for a

response, staring at the ceiling rather than risking looking at her doctor's face. "Anyway, from then on, I often didn't know what was true and what wasn't. It took a long time to decide how to answer questions teachers and parents tossed about so lightly. 'How was your day?' or 'Why did you do that?' or 'Why didn't you get the dust under the table if you swept?' Grown-ups didn't have the patience to wait for my answers. Since I was already guilty of untrustworthiness, I said whatever popped into my head and, of course, became guilty of lying."

When Lily paused for a moment, Dr. Woodling intervened. "That's a pretty powerful list. See if I caught all of it. Childish desire to explore, typical childish disobedience, intelligent but not having been taught writing, determined to be creative, losing self-control under stress, adolescent muscular strength beyond your expectation, anger with people who should have met your needs but didn't, and finally, trying to please and trying to grow up. Quite a list of indictments. Guess we better lock up the whole human race."

"They surely sound different when you describe them." Lily paused thoughtfully and then, with an impish grin, said, "But you must not forget my most flagrant sin—saving others when I can't save myself. Disturbed counselors are the most dangerous breeds walking the Earth."

"Especially when they're successful, huh? Traumatized girlfriend in high school feeling much happier. Seriously depressed friend with her college degree because of your influence. And two teens on this ward who were bears to live with when you were gone. Yeah, I guess you're dangerous."

Lily moaned, "Tell that to the nursing staff." Doctor and patient laughed together, and the laughter chased away the storm that threatened to follow self-disclosure. Even the volcanic rumblings could not shake the good earth.

"Lily, your guilt hangs entirely on that warped perception of yours, that set of condemning legalisms you formed at home, at church, and who knows where. Undo those rules. Accept your humanness. Accept your right to be bright and yet not all knowing. Accept your anger and use it. Crusade for social change, or religious reformation, or human rights. Anger does not preclude love. This Jesus you admire was an angry young man, but He was also known for His love for kids and sick people."

"Jesus, angry?"

"You think He whipped those temple storekeepers and drove a herd of cows out of the building with a sticky-sweet smile?"

"What? Oh, the cleansing of the temple. I guess He told off the religious leaders, too—snakes in the grass, whited sepulchers." Lily's eyes twinkled as she wished she could say such things to certain religious leaders in her past.

"I don't know too much about that," Dr. Woodling insisted, "but I know you are human and the rest of us humans would like you to join us on Earth."

Lily allowed the invitation to penetrate the depths of her soul. Slowly, she smiled. "I am! I really am human! I didn't really murder anyone. And by sixth grade I was so mixed-up that I didn't know what was happening."

"And because at one moment you showed a human quality like misunderstanding or disobedience does not mean that you are forever victim of that trait."

"Then I think I will accept your invitation. I'd consider it an honor to join you and the human race.

CHAPTER 15—THE ERUPTION
October 1968

    Lily expected her old patterns and fears to slough off like dead skin. She did not count on the fact that new skin must first replace the old or a sore results. Consequently, the harder she worked with Dr. Woodling and the more old beliefs and feelings she discarded, the more the volcano within her boiled. Often she felt compelled to quell its eruption by externalizing the turbulence in the form of matches or burning twists of paper. At Dr. Willoughby's insistence, Lily attempted to substitute a less dangerous release—banging a wet towel against the plastic seats of chairs stored in the vacant room at the far end of the main corridor.

    One evening following a particularly difficult day, Lily felt the internal pressure mounting. None of the medical students she trusted were on duty. Dr. Willoughby was away at a convention. And worst of all, the head nurse on duty was a soft, plump, ineffective woman who feared violence and hated Lily's disruption of the "good kitty" ward routine. Lily now had a roommate, a university student, and a scrawny girl who paced the halls and addressed everyone in an irritating, staccato voice. The previous night, that roommate had made a bid for the ward status of *most disturbed*, preventing Lily from sleeping in her own room. All day the lack of sleep and the challenge to Lily's dominance on the ward had fed the rumbling volcano.

    As Lily sensed her muscles tensing and watched the gray fog with its purple-black swirls of clouds descending, she realized something of previously unknown force was upon her. Instinctively she felt she must preserve her recently gained self-respect, must protect herself from the prying eyes of any ward member who might condemn. She raced to the door of her room and mutely motioned for Bonnie to keep everyone away. To hold the door closed, she formed a doorstop with her bed bolsters. With a wet towel, Lily beat out her fury on couches, pillows, and walls.

The world went black, then fiery red. Driven by the fury of the internal volcanic storm, her physical body propelled itself like a missile out of control. Twice Lily realized she was wildly hurtling around the room, bounding off walls, window screens, and the tops of desks.

Somehow Lily heard her roommate's shrill voice, "It's my room and I'm going in." In terror, Lily registered that it was not safe for them to be in the room together. As the door squeaked open, Lily rushed past the girl, turning in the direction of the vacant meeting room. There she could close the door and not be a spectacle.

Slamming the conference room door, Lily shoved chair after chair in its direction. Banging the towel, hitting her head on the wall, and hurling herself onto the radiator and into the window, Lily let the volcano erupt. To her horror, the door swung open and the head nurse's fat form stoppered it. Was it a hallucination or was she really there? Lily had no time to decide. She screamed her warning.

"Get out; get out; I'll kill you."

"No, you won't," the nurse muttered indolently.

Lily's hands contacted an armchair which soared through the air toward the figure. The apparition disappeared. Lily timed a steady beat with the towel on the seat of a chair. As the energy dissipated, Lily knelt, pounding her fists against the plastic seat. A figure—tall, white—loomed behind her. Ghost? No. Loving. Unafraid. Dr. Nunez. The resident who did not condemn.

Dr. Nunez was speaking to her in a low voice, calmly, insistently. Lily must walk down the hall to the lounge to get her regular medication. The thought of trying to navigate the hall, undulating like a heat wave in the desert, terrified Lily. Even if Dr. Nunez could prevent her from injuring anyone on the long trek, he could not still the savagely waving corridor. Lily tried to refuse, but the doctor's will was stronger than hers. Stiff-legged, arms interlocked behind her, eyes frozen in place, she shuffled toward the medicine cart.

As the worthless pills trickled down her throat, a nurse crooned, "There—there, you will feel better now." Another lie-- the medicine was so weak that its only effect was dizziness. But no point in arguing—no one believes a crazy woman.

Back in the vacant room with Dr. Nunez gone, Lily started beating the towel again with newly rising heat. A large orderly appeared in the doorway, a sentinel sent to observe but not to relieve the nameless torment with any real protection. Lily would not be watched.

She retreated to her bathroom, pulled out the hidden matches, and lost herself in their flame. No one interfered. Now that she no longer disrupted the ward's shining façade, the staff gladly forgot her. On that night, Lily inflicted upon her feelingless flesh the only deep burns she ever received—and no one knew.

At midnight, sitting wrapped in a blanket on her bed, Lily grumbled, "Some protection." And deep down she feared that, as Dr. Willoughby seemed to be wrong about the protection, she was also wrong about the other good things she had promised. Lily left for the Island.

After Lily's display on the ward, she sensed increasingly that the nursing staff did not want her. The chief psychiatric resident let it be known that she would like to send all violent patients to the state hospital, knowing the message would reach Lily. Lily issued her own counter-threats toward the chief resident's person and possessions. Fortunately, Dr. Willoughby intervened. Yet in the midst of the open warfare, Lily felt a growing strength and siding with reality. She constantly tested her new vigor and independence against the established system.

No longer allowed freedom to roam the grounds alone, Lily chose the escorted group walks as a prime target to measure her new strength. The distance she could trot off from the group without fear and in direct challenge of staff wishes marked the quantity and quality of her new self-assertion. This maneuver also indicated her respect or contempt for the staff members escorting the tour. The more secure she felt with the staff member, the more she challenged his control.

Her personal triumph came when she eluded Perky Perkitts and, totally leaving the group, escorted herself to the staff cafeteria to get a Coke. She reappeared on the ward a half hour later and, to the chagrin of the nurses, even their condemnation could not penetrate her rebellious smile of self-approval. From that point on, group walks were a game of cat-and-mouse, until finally Lily simply assigned herself the privilege of walking without supervision on the hospital grounds whenever the ward doors happened to be unlocked. After all, she reasoned, she would have to defy the system when she left the ward. She might as well get in practice.

During this period of challenge and revolt, Lily was assigned a new roommate, a timid seventeen-year-old, whose slight ninety-eight pounds and inarticulate backwoods ways were no match for Lily's muscular build and razor-edged tongue. But somehow the younger girl's vulnerability and ignorance of life outside her mountain hollow called forth the teacher in Lily. . Night after night Lily quelled her own pain and ignored the chiding nurses to reach out to this sallow-eyed girl. Day after day, Lily led, pleaded, and taught her roommate the best she knew of life. Discovering that she had a brilliant pupil, Lily risked interceding for the girl with the social worker, doctors, nurses, anyone who would listen and who might offer her roommate a hope and a future.

Lily's new health asserted itself in other ways. Since the night of the volcanic eruption, Lily's face had gained expressiveness and vitality, as though the force of the explosion had blasted away the old stony mask. Her gait acquired a swinging grace that replaced the jerky awkwardness of the past year. When she informed Dr.

Woodling that she would soon be leaving the ward, he was pleased.

One thing was needed—a place to go. Lily wanted to see her mother in hope that, after months apart and with the doctor's explanations, home would be ready to accept her, or she would have the strength to deal with the old home. Lily telephoned her parents. Her father was in the hospital again, but her mother would fly down.

Lily had hoped beyond hope that her mother would relate to her as an adult with a life and personality of her own. Dr. Willoughby arranged a conference between Lily's mother and the staff in an attempt to introduce Mrs. Farmer to the real Lily. But, confronted with unfamiliar emotional territory and confused by a few ill-worded questions, Mrs. Farmer felt hurt and abused, and the conference ran aground. At the end of her mother's visit, Lily commented to Dr. Woodling, "Since I'm no longer a model child, I'm just her spoiled little girl. To her, that is all I will ever be."

Thinking she had no choice but to remain in the university town, Lily received permission to search for work during the day. She consulted with the vocational rehabilitation counselor who, though friendly, offered no concrete assistance in locating a job. Lily applied at the university office, but her record counted against her there. Finally, she gathered courage and walked the mile to the Baptist hospital, combating her fear that an unknown monster hid behind each bush and that each car approaching her on the street would leap onto the sidewalk to crush her.

At the Baptist hospital, Lily marveled that the personnel lady seemed unaware of her sickness. The application form asked only about physical illness, and Lily did not mention that currently she was living on a psychiatric ward. She used Violet's address and phone number on the job application, assuming that her relative would not object.

Surprisingly, a ward clerk job on the evening shift would be available in two weeks. The pay was half of

Lily's salary as a lab assistant, but the job sounded easy. On the second interview, Lily was hired.

CHAPTER 16—MOVING THE MOUNTAIN
October 1968

Internally, Lily still quaked under her burden of guilt and fear. Panic often plummeted her out of the Earth-world onto the Island. In private, she banged her head and fought against the drawing power of fire. But outwardly Lily conformed to the ward expectations to be more sociable, non-violent, and nice. In the evenings, she gravitated to the clique of medical students who hung out in the ward lounge. To her delight, she was accepted as intelligent and knowledgeable. Only her own reticence prevented her from being "one of the boys"—her reticence and Lawrence Brigham.

Sexuality had been irrelevant to Lily. But Lawrence was different, not a boy playing at romance, but a mature man paying her thoughtful attention. Not "fresh" but openly friendly and complimentary, he extracted responses within her she had not known existed. With no experience, she fought the attraction by simple denial and temporarily succeeded in evading her feelings. Succeeded until on Sunday afternoon when Lawrence Brigham came alone to her room.

He came bearing what he thought was good news: he had received permission to remain on psychiatric rotation and take Lily as his patient. But what was good news to the doctor raised gale winds in the head of the patient. Lily had to fight the storm of terror—terror of her own confused impulses—to force a weak smile.

"Thank you, Lawrence, I appreciate your effort," she managed. But her head shouted, *Go away. Stay away. Don't make me face my female incompetency. I hate my body and its sensations. They confuse me. I don't know how to relate to men and I don't want to learn.*

Lily heard the rumble of distant thunder within her and trembled lest she be unable to hide the internal storm. Lawrence had cared enough to extend himself for her. She must not openly reject him.

Trying to balance between her rising terror and her desire to be polite, Lily asked uncertainly, "Lawrence, it has been a long day and I'm tired. Could I talk to you another time?"

Graciously Dr. Lawrence Brigham left, promising to see her that evening.

When he had gone, Lily tried to think, but the storm roared through her head. She paced the floor, battling the winds, searching for their origin. Her mind followed the swirling clouds out through the vast internal spaces until it saw red—the red of the volcano with steam pouring from it, transforming into the winds of the storm.

"The volcano, the lake of rage," Lily whispered to herself. "The gale comes from the lake of rage. Dr. Willoughby would ask why I am angry. I don't know."

As if in answer, the voice of the wind roared, *Thwarted. Guilty of hope and thwarted.* Then Lily knew. Dr. Willoughby had promised her a mature woman medical student to help Lily deal with her feelings about femaleness. Lily had counted on this woman as a new model to imitate. Now this promise would be denied.

"But that's not enough to arouse the volcano," she insisted.

Rude laughter rode in on the winds. Voices crackled, *Sinful, sexual, deluded, mocked.* Instantly she recognized the voices as those of the exiled priests of the Island. They continued, *We have you trapped this time. You are ours.* Lily was trapped for she felt she could never express herself to Dr. Brigham and would therefore be without relief or release. *Cursed and doomed,* the voices intoned. Cursed and doomed to infect those she loved with her rottenness. Dr. Willoughby had said that she was not contagious, but Dr. Willoughby had been wrong about the protection.

The gale, the rumbling volcano, and now rebellion on the Island. It was too much. She had to stop it before she lost all reason. She would pay the penalty while there was still time. Ritualistically, Lily repeated, "I will burn for my guilt," and added matter-of-factly, "and this time the guilt is real."

She had surrendered all the matches to Dr. Woodling, and matches were currently in short supply on the ward. But Bonnie, a heavy smoker, perpetually hid a book in her desk drawer. Lily sprinted across the hall toward Bonnie's room, almost colliding with Dr. Woodling.

"Where are you going in such a hurry?" he exclaimed as he dodged.

"Oh, uh, just to visit Bonnie. See you later." But the fire-wish had seeped out through her eyes.

Bonnie was out of her room. Quickly Lily grabbed the matches and skittered back to her own room. Disliking the act of theft, Lily decided to pay a little extra for that guilt.

In her bathroom with the door locked, she had lit only one match when she heard Dr. Woodling's heavy tread enter her room. "Lily, come out here." He suspected. Caught.

"Uh, just a minute." She made bathroom sounds while she found a hiding place for the matches.

"Lily, get out here *NOW*," he bellowed.

Lily came out, faking nonchalance yet yearning for him to penetrate her façade. The medical student had grown wise to Lily's inability to directly ask for help. "If the mountain won't come to Mohammed, then Mohammed will go to the mountain," he said matter-of-factly. "I got your message. Sit down. What are you upset about?"

Though she could not explain her feelings, the presence of the man who had so frequently forced his will over hers temporarily plugged the volcano. Without the volcano, the winds died.

"I can't tell you."

"After all this time, you don't trust me? I'm really a lousy doctor."

'No! You're good. But you're—a—a—a man."

"That's a crime? Look, is this connected with Dr. Brigham?"

"No." The truth was mortifying, but she could not lie to a person who had shared so much of himself. "Yes, it's Lawrence."

"Did he say something?"

"He's going to be my new student therapist. Dr. Willoughby promised me a woman to help my identity problem."

"If you mean feeling like a woman, I think Lawrence can handle that."

Lily reeled through her data bank but found no long-term evasion. If she could not confide in Dr. Woodling, she could never trust anyone. "That's the problem."

"Are you trying to say that you find Lawrence Brigham sexually attractive? He will be highly complimented. And you have good taste."

Lily turned pink, red, and purple—embarrassed, flabbergasted, and flattered. Dr. Woodling liked the idea! That Lawrence would be anything but insulted had never occurred to her. "But—but I'm a—a mental patient."

"You're an attractive young woman. I won't let you put yourself down."

"Attractive? Me?"

"Everyone has noticed except you. Look at yourself in the mirror."

"That's vain."

"That's self-respect and self-love."

Lily looked. The mask was gone. The once-frozen eyes danced with a hint of mischievousness. Her short chestnut hair waved and curled, shining in the sunlight. Her makeup needed attention, but the face underneath was sensitive and glowing. Lily smiled at herself, and then turned to Dr. Woodling. "What do I do?"

"I'm going to tell Dr. Brigham what you are feeling. He will handle the rest. Stay right here. Oh, is there something you want to give me?"

Lily grinned sheepishly and handed over the matches.

"You've outgrown the need for these," Dr. Woodling commented as he left the room.

When Lawrence Brigham settled himself on the couch opposite her, Lily intended to be demure. Lawrence Brigham upset her plan in one sentence. "Tell me how you feel about me—what you like, dislike, and why."

Lily had never told any man that she liked him. She had verbalized hate but not attraction. Slowly, painfully, she described how she valued Lawrence's acceptance and compliments. Then she described his dark, pool-like eyes, the long, graceful lashes, the peculiar twist of his lips about his cherry-stemmed pipe, and finally his deep voice that resounded like music from every corner of the room. That Lawrence carried a force field of secure excitement, she could not explain.

"I want you to like me, and I'm afraid you won't." Lily had never asked to be liked. She listened for the head winds to whip into a gale. Silence!

"I asked to take on an extra assignment because I find you ugly, clumsy, and offensive? Lily, I'm flattered by your attention. Would I be out of line to say that I find you good company? You're sharp, well read. You have a quick, sensitive disposition and are capable of much love. And if I may say so without seeming fresh, you're pretty."

"Not fresh. Just a liar," Lily quipped defensively.

"Is it so devastating to be a responsive woman attracted to the opposite sex? Is that evil?"

Lily struggled. Her early church and home training shouted, *yes*. Echoes of Pastor David insisted, *No, that is good;* and her own sensations cast their weight with Pastor David. She grinned. "No, that's good. I'm human and real."

"My objective for the next eight weeks is for you to learn to enjoy life and appreciate yourself."

Lily paled. Enjoyment and appreciation were ominous strangers.

"You look uncertain," Dr. Brigham observed.

"Joy has a terrible price. Play your flute and pay the piper."

"That is your old fantasy world. In the real world, happiness doesn't bring pain. You don't have to accept that old pattern of punishment now. It's your choice."

"A choice? Maybe. At least not to pay the price in the old sense. But to love is to be hurt by the world. Don't tell me differently."

"It depends on what we do with our love, with whatever happens in our lives. Lily, you can choose to act, rather than react. You don't have to follow a programmed script. If I hurt you, you don't have to run away and turn against yourself and me. You can be openly angry. Or you can confront me with logic. Or you can make a joke of it."

"The other side is that I don't want to hurt you. People I love always get hurt."

"You mean that rottenness of yours? I'm not subject to your control. I act, not react. So you can't spoil me."

"But it's contagious, just being close to me."

"I'm not afraid. In fact I want to escort you on a walk after supper. You would enjoy getting out of this stuffy building, wouldn't you?"

"I might get upset or violent."

"So hit me. I don't break. I've done my share of fighting and played a bit of football." Lily gasped. "Well, come here and hit me and see."

At the mental picture of her feeble right hook against the muscular biceps, Lily burst into laughter. "Okay, okay, I get the message. You can take care of yourself. So I trust you. Lawrence, you're terrific."

During the next week, Lawrence was Lily's friend and companion introducing her to a sweeter reality. Meanwhile, Dr. Woodling drove Lily mercilessly in their analysis of her family, pushing to complete the project before the end of his psychiatric service. The interview with Mrs. Farmer had given Dr. Woodling new ammunition. He forced Lily to examine incident after incident in which her mother's well-meaning protection had played into Lily's distorted perceptual system.

Lily summarized their discussions. "I guess the whole business started because I wanted to be normal, like all the other kids. But home, school, and church said, 'That's wrong.' I couldn't live by the double standard. I couldn't play the game of deceit. I chose to be a doll for the adults to admire, a puppet programmed with computer perfection.

"Then I didn't fit with the other children. Lonely, I made up my own friends, established my own set of rules based on those old legalisms, and the illness was off and running. All along—even now—my plea is, 'Let me be me. Value me. Approve my strengths and don't protect my weaknesses.' I must have a fantastically strong will to have fought for my independence all these years when I didn't really believe I even had the right to be."

"What do you think was the greatest source of your distortions?"

"My church!"

Dr. Woodling winced. He had expected the pat answer, *home*.

"My parents made the emotional quagmire. My body contributed its general havoc. But the church dealt out the neurotic guilt, the false expectations of the world and myself, the indefinable fears of my natural drives, and the thrice-weekly authoritative condemnations. I don't know if I can ever attend a church of that denomination that preaches such negative emotions again. Now that I know you and Lawrence and the other guys here, I see the world differently, and I just don't like most Christians I've known."

Dr. Woodling sat stunned. No one had intended to destroy Lily's religious faith, only to make her well.

Lily clarified the issue. "Dr. Woodling, don't misunderstand. I love Jesus. He is my best Friend. The healthier I become, the more clearly I know Him and love Him. My decision to live in reality was for His sake. But Jesus has little relationship to the church that I grew up in. My faith isn't in a group of people: it's in God."

November-December 1968

With the assistance of Dr. Willoughby and the medical students, Lily planned her immediate future. She would live on the ward for the first week of her new job at the Baptist hospital. If all went well, Lily would then temporarily move to her Aunt Violet's house until she found an apartment. She could spend her mornings on the ward to occupy her free time and provide a bit of nostalgic reassurance. On occasion, she might be able to take her friends for short trips. Both Lawrence and the woman student promised by Dr. Willoughby would be her therapists, one to encourage and support, the other to dissect and challenge.

On the appointed day, Lily reported to her new job. On the next appointed day, she moved from the ward. On the surface, life was fine. Only her so-called histrionic performances, when she returned to the ward demanding her doctors, betrayed the terror she grappled with moment by moment. Many of the nursing staff effectively communicated their annoyance with her outbursts and her presence on the ward.

If they only knew the fear I fight. If they understood the immense vastness of time/space to be crossed just to propel myself through their world, just to insure hearing and vision and reasonableness. They never feel the effort to smile, to be alert, to control body and tongue on the job. Well, allow them their humanness.

By the end of the first two weeks of freedom, Lily felt herself sinking. Physically the structure of life was too uncertain—food, water, bathrooms, and traffic—all were unpredictable and protection was nonexistent. Though her job was simple, it contained hidden rules of interpersonal relationships that were too vague for Lily's infant grasp of reality. She yearned for more structure and familiar activity.

Her systematic mind studied new strategies for security. At the end of this student rotation, Lily would be without a therapist whom she knew. She would quit her job and go home. At least the home terrors were familiar and physical environment more definable.

After Christmas, she would enroll in this university in special education. Dr. Willoughby had said that Lily should be able to teach, and Lily had enjoyed her previous work with slower-moving handicapped children.

Though she wanted her plans to remain a secret, she needed assistance to gain immediate admission to graduate school. Knowing her woman therapist's influence in the education department, Lily convinced herself to ask for help. To her surprise, both her therapist and Dr. Willoughby recommended her to the special education department, and Lily was accepted.

CHAPTER 17–THE UNIVERSITY
January 1969

On January 6, Lily Farmer entered university life as a graduate student in special education. Following her carefully planned strategy, she had resigned her job, had returned home for Christmas, and now assigned herself to what she supposed was a structured environment.

College life, as Lily had known it previously, had provided food, shelter, friends, and a regimentation of personal conduct that created a measure of security. In her undergraduate days, someone had always known where she was, if she was missing, whether she was eating properly, if she was ill. The distance between buildings was minimal, but if she momentarily lost her direction, she could usually follow an acquaintance going to the same building. Patterns of life—dress, thought, rising and bedtime, and special activities—had been relatively uniform for all students, and Lily needed only to drift with the stream.

But the university had no stream. An enormous, open society with as many life-styles as students, the university demanded independence and presence of mind. It was a ten-minute walk across open, unguarded spaces from Lily's dormitory to the central cafeteria. Once there, Lily was faced with a myriad of choices among foods, choices requiring rapid-fire decisions impossible to Lily's fear-burdened mind. Often she carried her tray to a table, only to discover she had two meats, no vegetables, and a gooey dessert that would stick in her throat. Even more often she ate alone. Though at first she invited herself into small groups already at the tables in anticipation of making friends, she soon discovered that the same group was never present at the next meal and her forced amiability had been wasted.

Alone too she tackled the unpredictable journeys between classes, often afraid of an unseen assailant lurking behind a tree, constantly wondering if she would reach her next class or be lost forever. The distance from her special education class to her sociology class required that she walk halfway across campus in ten minutes. For other students, the route posed no threat: the university was small by national standards and the sidewalks were well marked. But in Lily's disoriented state, the route seemed to change daily. Buildings cropped up where parking lots should have been; hedges sprang up where she expected to cut across a grassy lawn. Regardless of how doggedly she persisted in her goal, Lily rarely arrived at class on time, and in sociology, part of her grade depended on punctuality.

The tremendous expanse of time unoccupied by classes or formal activities also troubled Lily. At her undergraduate school, the bulk of her day was planned for her, and the rest was required for homework. But at the university, classes met only a few hours a week and the assignments were so simple that Lily needed little time for their completion. How she spent the remainder of her day no one knew or cared.

In His mercy, God provided Lily with a sip of success, a vinegar sponge on the cross of loneliness. Because of her excellent academic record and through Dr. Willoughby's influence, Lily was awarded an assistantship in the special education materials center. When the six graduate assistants were assigned the basement of the old brick building as their office, Lily unobtrusively took up residence. If the materials center was open, Lily could be found in the basement. There she knew she must keep up a façade of normalcy, and the knowledge defended her against the tempest howling within her.

Her supervisor in the materials center seemed oblivious of Lily's condition and assigned her task upon responsible task. To Lily's delight, she discovered that her orderly mind was ideal for the library resource work. She became master keeper of all files; if any book, catalog, or information temporarily eluded the regular staff, their immediate response was, "Ask Lily. She'll know." Her supervisor generously doled out the praise that Lily's success-starved being craved. Lily responded by even more lively involvement in the center's functions, which in turn spiraled into more success.

On weekends, Lily sought solace from the ambiguity of campus life at her Aunt Violet's. A former army nurse, Violet treated Lily's peculiarities as merely part of a unique personality, as legitimate as the individualistic personalities of her own five children. Yet when Lily blurted out excerpts from her unending list of confusions, Violet responded with an alert, empathetic ear, totally accepting, uncannily practical. Violet's daughters included Lily in their activities and brought fun and new healthy patterns into her life. Each Monday when she had to return to the emptiness of the university, Lily yearned silently, *if only I could stay with Violet forever, I would be free.*

February 1969

Lost in a campus life beyond her comprehension, Lily sunk lower into depression and hopelessness. A month after she had returned to the university, Lily discovered that Dr. Willoughby no longer supervised her case, and that the new psychiatrist was the old troll who had sent her back to the Christian college, decreeing her a waste of time. The new doctor's theory was that Lily's illness was self-induced and could be quickly remedied by a "relationship" with an overpowering male.

In protest, Lily wrote to Dr. Willoughby, hoping somehow that the psychiatrist would come to her aid. Dr. Willoughby's reply by letter caringly but firmly informed Lily that university clinic policy prohibited her intervention in outpatient affairs.

Lily dared not assert her need again. Reeling under the impact of this abandonment, Lily arrived at her night class, Development of Human Potential. Usually she looked forward to this class composed of older students, most of them practicing professionals who liked and respected her. To compensate for her inexperience, Lily had thrown all of her intellectual prowess into the intense class discussions and had gained a place of prominence. A group of eight social workers had asked her to join them in demonstrating the dynamics of an encounter group, a currently popular form of self-exploration.

Lily had looked forward to the adventure. But tonight as she surveyed the passive faces of students in the large circle of chairs around the room, Lily was terrified. Thirty pairs of well-trained eyes would be watching her, observing her for flaws. What would they see? Would she be able to sustain her reputation as an intellectual? Would she be able to prevent Jerry, the perceptive leader, from penetrating her carefully constructed exterior and discovering the stench of the illness inside? She had rejoiced that no one in class knew she was "schizie", but, as she took her seat with the demonstration group in the center of the room, she sensed the likelihood of exposure and trembled.

Jerry started the session by playing a tape recording on the merits of being real, of allowing people to know one's true self. Lily's mind grappled with the possibility that maybe here the real Lily would be accepted. But just as quickly, from her Island home deep inside, she heard her big brother shouting, *No, Lily, don't expose yourself. Keep your mask on. Be careful.*

When the recording stopped, Jerry paired off the group members and explained the procedure. Each group member would tell his partner how he felt about that person. That partner and other group members were expected to respond and to respond in terms of honest feelings, not thoughts. Jerry asked two women who were co-workers at a social service agency to demonstrate the procedure. After that, the pairs took turns. Class comments were basically positive and suggestions helpful.

Yet, for Lily, the pressure mounted. People were

watching, expecting her to respond. But respond in what way? The name of the game was emotional honesty, but Lily knew her emotions were not socially acceptable. What to say? How to smile?

At that moment of doubt, Jerry intruded. "Lily, how do you feel about what I just said?"

Lost to what had just occurred, Lily hedged. "Interesting. Very interesting."

"That's a thought. Not a feeling. How do you feel about my criticizing Maria? She is your partner."

"I don't feel" Lily said, then hastily covered, "I mean I feel you have a right to your own opinion."

"Lily, you tell Maria how you feel about her and she will respond."

Lily admired Maria, a black school social worker, but as she began to explain that admiration, she saw her own words written in the air, each word with a pair of wings. *The meanings. They are threatening to fly away.* Lily cringed visibly. *I won't be able to understand anymore. Oh, no!*

"What is the matter, Lily?" Jerry probed. "Is it hard to directly tell someone you like her?"

Jerry was right. She had idolized Dr. Willoughby, and Dr. Willoughby had deserted her. She was now complimenting Maria; she would be rejected again. As fast as the realization flitted through Lily's consciousness, she pushed it down into the lower regions.

"No, it's not that. It's nothing. Maria, your turn."

Lily stared at the words hanging in the air, stared with her eyes at the vision in her mind. *The wings, they are flapping.* Above the wings ran a line of musical notes. *Laughter. I'm going to laugh. No, I mustn't. Lily, don't laugh. Just smile pleasantly at Maria.* The notes danced up and down. The wings flapped.

"In general, Lily," Maria was concluding, "I feel you are a wholesome girl, bright, friendly, with much to offer the class. But you seem to live inside a shell. I would like to know you better."

Manic laughter reverberated through the room, rising from the depths of Lily's being, bursting from her wide-open mouth into the real world.

The laughter stopped. Lily gazed about her. She saw shapes, forms, people moving, mouths talking. But she understood nothing. The meaning of words and events had vanished.

An hour later, when she regained cloudy awareness, Lily was sitting at her regular desk in the classroom. In front of her on her notebook was scrawled, "The meanings have flown. For a moment I faced the truth. I risked myself before the group. The meanings danced to the music of my laugh. When the laughter shattered, the meanings scattered."

Mentally Lily blacked out. When she rejoined the real world, she was on her bed in her efficiency apartment in the university complex. Excruciating mental pain wracked every fiber of her consciousness. Inexorable pressure inside her threatened to force the blood through her skin, to atomize her whole being, sending each particle a separate direction throughout the entire universe so that no evidence of a human being remained.

Lily shrieked, "God, help me. I'm going to disintegrate."

She curled into a ball on her bed and held herself tightly until the light of morning signaled the necessity for activity. Aching, stiff, weak, she arose. "Breakfast, I have to go to breakfast. Then comes class. Then lunch, then work, then supper. Then night. Night—I will not spend another like the past few. I will acknowledge my guilt. We will see."

Night came. As always, Lily was alone, alone with the inner torment of the living death. As though in a trance, she announced, "I am guilty. I liked Dr. Willoughby. I asked for help. I liked Maria. I had feelings. I am guilty." The admission released the volcanic rage inside her and her arms hurled the desk chair across the room. In desperation she ran to the tile and concrete bathroom. Grabbing her matches, she sought the release of fire, burning length upon length of toilet paper and toweling.

She craved seeing her dress ablaze, but she had promised Dr. Willoughby she would not burn herself again; she would not break that promise as long as reason lasted at all. Agitated, coughing, Lily stared into the flames, waiting for them to assuage her torment. But this night, even the flames withheld their comfort. And the campus police who drove frequently past her window did not notice the irregular flashes of light. Dr. Willoughby was wrong; even the police did not always come.

Lily's inner turmoil propelled her through useless, ceaseless motion for the next two days. Thursday night she craved sleep. With no other relief at hand, she consumed a harmlessly low overdose of her weak tranquilizers and a dozen aspirin. She was familiar with the chemistry of tranquilizers and knew she had not taken enough to do permanent damage. She waited for sleep. But an unexpected and irresistible fear caught her instead, propelling her to the hospital emergency room for help. Instead of the comfort, release, and acceptance she yearned for, there she met stomach pumps and IV's administered with a vengeance. Finally, with a dose of ipecac, she was sent home to vomit and excrete alone. The message: "You are a pain; don't bother us."

During the next month and a half, whenever the volcano spewed out its memories, taunts, and guilt, Lily's behavior was erratic and, in private, violent. Her screams and the crash of glasses seemed bound in by her own apartment walls, however, for no one ever answered and no one in the building offered to be her friend.

March-April 1969

Without Dr. Willoughby, therapy degenerated into a farce, a play with Lily as the villain whose symbolic hysterics were not understood by the medical students. The troll-like psychiatrist made her dislike of Lily quite clear. Twice Lily went to the emergency room in hope of finding one of the residents she had known on the ward, but she was met with an attitude that said, "We are not supposed to treat you. You just want attention. Go home and behave yourself."

In spite of the torments, Lily studied diligently and worked hard at her job in the materials center. The job increased in complexity. Lily felt her understanding unequal to the tasks, but, as long as her supervisor continued to assign her work in full confidence of her ability to perform, Lily continued to try.

Finally the day came when even the solace of work was denied her. On a departmental outing, Lily was suddenly overwhelmed by inexplicable fear. She turned to the graduate assistant next to her, one she ventured to call *friend*.

"I'm scared. It hurts so badly. I'd rather die than go on living this way." The girl recoiled in horror. Lily was mentally gone.

The next day, Lily was summoned to the office of the head of the department. Under his probing, she admitted that she constantly fought against emotional pain and violence, but she insisted the professor should have known. Dr. Willoughby had contacted him before her admission to the program. She could still function; she had to function. The department head ignored her rationale and coolly informed her that she was unfit to teach children; therefore she need not return the next semester.

In her journal that evening Lily wrote: "April 30, 1969. Be honest—get punished! When I am honest, I get punished. I was honest about my background, about my feelings, and now, no assistantship, no program, no recommendation. I was honest, and a door banged in my face. On the ward, I was honest about my feelings. I admitted that I burned for my guilt. I lost privileges. Punished.

"Punished or protected? The ward people said *protected* from situations that would hurt me. The department head said the same thing. Are they just excusing their actions? Or is protection just another name for punishment?"

CHAPTER 18—LIMBO
June 1969

   Lily's ejection from the university thrust her back into her parents' home. Mrs. Farmer forced a tense, motherly attitude to disguise the aching disillusionment in her heart. Mr. Farmer occupied Lily with physical work and insisted she was normal—just having a little trouble growing up. Though Lily thrived on her parents' attention for the first few weeks, ancient shadows of confusion and condemnation lurked among the all-too-familiar walls, walls of both physical and social isolation
   At expense thoroughly beyond their means, the Farmers admitted Lily as a patient to a church-related psychiatric clinic and day treatment center. Lily stayed with a foster family during the week, attended the day treatment center, and returned home on weekends. She marveled that the older couple with whom she stayed behaved as if she were acceptable, real, with a right to be herself. Her sickness seemed irrelevant.
   At the day treatment center, the recreation and new friendships with other patients eased her inner loneliness for the first three weeks, but, as the novelty wore away, the inevitable nameless fears and aggression again asserted themselves. The clinic staff, more interested in keeping the peace than in dealing with the underlying disorder, refused to do open warfare for Lily against her inner storms. Their concept of therapy far exceeded Lily's meager grasp of the laws of social reality.
   Intending to mobilize her strongest defense against her illness, her relationship with God, Lily sought out the chaplain. Ignoring Lily's feelings of helplessness against the whirling chaos inside her, the chaplain parroted the hardline theology that Lily must change herself; God would

not change her. When he continued with the declaration that he did not accept all of the Bible as God's true Word, Lily inwardly shut up her longings, her questions, her love into a remote corner of her being and slammed the door, determined never to be hurt again by the clinic staff. Outwardly she merely excused herself from the chaplain's office. Now, with both love and logic locked away and useless, violence erupted against the clinic as a last desperate plea. The plea went unheard. Lily left the clinic in bitterness.

During the next three years, Lily lived in limbo. She worked a year as a counselor at a church-sponsored correctional school. Then, driven by restless loneliness, she quit her job and enrolled as a graduate student in a small Catholic college in a city near her parents' home.

On Saturdays, her mother drove Lily to the state capitol for expensive therapy with a private Christian psychiatrist. The psychiatrist was caring and listened carefully and empathically. His approach was entirely different than anything Lily had previously experienced. He regarded Lily's pathology as a combination between a medical problem and a lack of social skills. First, he prescribed a low dosage of a traditional antipsychotic medication with which Lily was familiar from her high school paper on tranquilizers. Lily found the medication took the edge off the irrational anger so that she could think more clearly.

Then the psychiatrist began teaching Lily to use her cognitive skills to analyze social situations, to focus on thoughts rather than feelings. Through the sessions, Lily discovered what Lawrence Brigham had once told her: that, for any one situation, there were numerous possible ways to respond. She had legitimate choices. She was not helplessly locked into one set of predetermined reactions: she could use her good mind to think of new and more productive, even enjoyable, ways to respond. Furthermore, she need not be the victim when confronted by conflicting belief systems and contradictory authorities. She could assert her own beliefs and state her own position: that was not being arrogant or sinfully proud, as she had been taught subtly. "What I've learned from this psychiatrist," Lily wrote in her journal, "is that it is all right to stand up for myself and how to do that creatively."

With this discovery, Lily's self control stabilized and her exterior surface appeared more normal. Her thinking seemed more logical, less laced with expressions unintelligible to other people. But Lily knew that mental health was more than the absence of observable sickness, and that the healthy processes in her were no more developed than when Lawrence Brigham had first escorted her into the social world. Lily marked time, waiting for death or complete insanity, whichever came first.

From the three aimless years between 1969 and 1972, four events carved permanent impressions into Lily's being.

October 1969

The first event occurred during the summer after she moved home from the university, before her job began at the correctional school. Since her break with Prof Filbert, Lily had struggled with a burden of doubt and conflict about God, the Church, and Christianity. If only she could understand and conquer these conflicts, Lily felt she would have a firm base for solving her other problems.

Her search led her to return to her former home church where her parents were still active. Lily thought that the new pastor, who was young and well educated, could understand her plight and clear away the entangling cobwebs of theological jargon and direct her towards the freedom that Christ promised but that she did not experience.

For hours, Lily visited with his wife, played with his small children, and discussed with the pastor the realms of the spirit and the mind. If Lily's social perception had been sharper, the pastor's sly barbs concerning the inferiority of women and the fate of young rebels would have alerted her. But in naïve hopefulness, Lily trusted too far. She asked to appear before the examining board of the church to be readmitted to church membership.

One Sunday after the worship service, Lily strode confidently into the basement office, with its cold gray concrete block walls and cement floor, to meet with the church board. Casually she seated herself on a metal folding chair before the three men, expecting a friendly chat, a pat on the back, and a glad-to-have-you-with-us-again. She smiled cheerfully at the men—her former high school teacher; a long-time family friend; and the young pastor. All the men had heard Lily's frequent expression of her love for Jesus; all knew that she had endured some sort of trauma; all had seen her kindness and gentleness with children in the church. She had no thought other than that she could trust these men.

Her high school teacher began. "Lily, we understand that you want to be reinstated as a member of this church. You had changed your membership to a different denomination while you were away. Is that right?"

"Yes, I joined the church that was part of the college I attended. Now I'm back here living with my parents, so I should be part of this church again."

"Very well. I see." The teacher shifted uneasily in his chair and looked down at a typed page on his lap. "Because that church is theologically liberal, it is necessary for us to ask you some questions."

Perplexed but not alarmed, Lily nodded and smiled. "Okay."

The teacher raised the printed sheet and read the first question. "Do you accept Jesus Christ as personal Savior and Redeemer from your sins, without whom you are totally and hopelessly lost?"

Lily was lost, but only in the verbiage. "I don't use those terms," she tried to explain honestly. "Savior and Redeemer have no meaning for me in everyday life. I want my Christianity to be real. Jesus is my Best Friend."

Glances sailed from her teacher to the other men.

Lily sensed tension that she could not understand. Then the man who had been a friend of her family, who had eaten at their table, whom Lily would have trusted with her life, read the next question. "Do you believe that immersion is the only scripturally-prescribed mode of baptism and rejection thereof constitutes rejection of God's commands? Have you obeyed that commandment?"

Why are they asking what they already know? Lily thought. *They know I was immersed in this church. Maybe they want to know how I see baptism now that I've had more experiences.* With the same candor that had endeared her to her medical student therapists, Lily answered, "I have been immersed, and it was a terrifying experience. I was seven years old, and I almost drowned. Some of the most Spirit-filled people I know have not been immersed. Considering how God works through them, He must not be too worried about how you are baptized."

Words whizzed through the room like arrows—comments concerning ecumenical apostates and reminders of the doom of young ladies who dared to lift themselves up in the face of Almighty God. Lily did not understand. Her mind clouded and fog settled before her eyes. Through the fog, Lily saw the pastor leaning toward her, his usual amiable grin replaced by a strange hawkish expression.

His question was currently explosive among theologians. "Do you believe in the verbal plenary inspiration of the Scriptures and in inerrancy and infallibility thereof? Do you subscribe to the literal method of interpretation?"

From years of training in Sunday school, Lily knew the expected answer but she was not willing to lie. "I believe the Bible says what it means and means what it says. I don't use those theological terms to describe normal life, and I don't use them to describe the Bible. Every scholar I know of attaches a different meaning to them, and I won't fasten my faith to a dispute." Lily's indignation began to rise; her vision cleared; her green eyes snapped; her voice acquired a sharp edge. As she looked around at the faces she had thought were friends, her emotions overcame reason. "And if by literal interpretation, if you mean using the Bible as a weapon, verse by verse, NO!"

The agitation in the room had set the gale winds howling in Lily's head; fighting their verbal blasts against her rationality, and keeping herself in her seat required boundless courage and determination. Blinded by the storm of tightly controlled emotions in the room, neither Lily nor the board members realized that the conflict was not in important differences of belief but in the use of words.

Like a grand inquisitor about to pass sentence, the pastor demanded, "And will you submit to the authority of the officers of this church, live by its laws and restrictions, and follow its precepts?"

This had gone too far. In spite of the storm in her emotions, Lily straightened rigidly erect, fully alert, calling on her academic prowess in an effort to balance respect for the authority of the church with expression of her own studied convictions and integrity. Into her mind came a saying of an old saint and prayer warrior whom she had admired in college years. "Sirs," Lily pronounced with conviction, "I take my orders from Headquarters. I am a slave to no man."

The pastor rose, shaking his head in mock sympathy. He had held the power to save Lily from agony, to rephrase the questions into normal English, to interpret her answers with consideration and love. Instead, he had ordered and led the inquisition. Now he wanted to appear noble, benevolent, and innocent. With a triumphant gleam in his eye, he stood over Lily. "I'm sorry, Lily. I don't believe you belong in our congregation. I hope someday you will see the error of your ways."

Lily rose quickly and stood at military attention, facing him: then looking each man in the eye, she said, "I do *not* belong in this congregation of legalists and Pharisees. My Jesus is love and mercy and peace. He called your kind 'snakes in the grass' and 'whitewashed graves.' You can keep your church. Good-bye."

Minutes later, when Lily met her parents in the vestibule, Mrs. Farmer started to ask her about the meeting, but Lily cut her off with a heart-freezing stare, and said coldly, "I should have known what they are. I'm going to the car and I won't be back."

Though Lily had shown no pain or fear before the church leaders, the deep agony of their betrayal and condemnation festered for months. The wounds so self-righteously inflicted by those whom she should have been able to trust confirmed Lily's former suspicions. Authorities, especially Christian authorities, were either incompetent or malicious. She granted them the benefit of being incompetent.

Lily pleaded with God for death.

November 1969—June 1970

Instead of death, God sent a rare old evangelist, a gentle-faced man with hair thinning and back bent from years carrying others' burdens. His simple tactics were love and respect. Rev. Dopson sacrificed many evenings to sit with Lily on her parents' glassed-in porch and explain Scripture with love, rather than with law. Looking out through the windows at the beauties of nature, he talked about God who is powerful enough to create each leaf, each star, and loving enough to come once in history to live with us, as Jesus, and take the punishment that we deserve. The evangelist spoke of Lily's suffering as bringing her closer to Jesus. He affirmed Lily's gift of praying, already knowing that what she asked was God's will and would be granted. He called this quality "the prayer of faith." When Lily confided that Jesus spoke to her in a voice that she heard, the wise man did not condemn her as deluded, but rejoiced in Christ's nearness.

Two years after Lily had given Dr. Willoughby her decision to live in reality, the night came in late spring when Lily faced herself squarely, knowing that her mind was again slipping beyond her control. Would she totally lose what she had gained of this precious reality? Was she cursed to eternal cycles of disintegration? How could Jesus ever use her? How could God ever fulfill the promise latent in her natural talents? Lily phoned Rev. Dopson. Though he had just returned from a prolonged tour and was weary, he came.

As they sat together on the back porch, Lily gazed for a few moments at the stars spattering the dark sky, and then at the lined face of the pastor, now softened by the yellow light overhead. With efforts, she began, "Reverend Dopson, I love Jesus. I stayed alive for Him. I want more than anything else to witness and live for Him. But I can't. No one will listen to a girl who is periodically crazy."

The evangelist looked her straight in the eye, as though this were a perfectly normal conversation and said matter-of-factly, "Your God cannot use a mentally ill person? Mine can."

Rev. Dopson recounted case upon case in which God had worked through mental illness to reach into otherwise impenetrable circumstances. The final example was a lady who had lived most of her adult life in a state hospital. As long as she had that security and structure, she thrived, but in the outside world, she withered like a violet in the desert.

"Other pastors may consider this lady's life a waste, but I believe she was God's special flower," the evangelist said gently. "She could get emotionally close to patients that the staff could not reach. She could present the good news of Jesus' love to patients otherwise closed to the Gospel. Even the staff respected her faith, and some found Christ through her. God blessed her with a special ministry, and in Heaven she will have her reward." He smiled tenderly at Lily, and she saw the love of Christ in his eyes and light shining from his face.

"Lily, God knows how much you have suffered. He knows your dedication to Him. Trust God's opinion of you. Perhaps now He offers one final point of surrender. If God wants you to be mentally ill all of your life in order to use you in His service, are you willing?"

Lily swallowed hard. She saw the choice. She knew the

price. She forced her mind to listen for Jesus' voice. He was silent. Lily must choose independently—her will or total surrender to God at any price.

"I promised Jesus I would follow Him anywhere when I was in high school. I meant it. If it is His will that I be mentally ill all of my life, I am ready. Could we please pray? I need Him NOW." Sobs punctuated her speech as she called out to her beloved Friend. "It's all right, Jesus, if that's what You want. But don't let me dishonor You when I am confused. Be close to me. I love You. "

Rev. Dopson prayed. Then together they shared Lily's decision with her parents. Setting aside their hurt and pride, Mr. and Mrs. Farmer committed Lily totally to God's will. For the first time in years, Lily's love for her parents flowed freely and smoothly. They loved her enough to let her belong to Jesus, to let her go. What more could she ask? The hate she had never wanted to feel melted into the warm breeze and disappeared forever.

September 1970

The third was a double event that opened Lily to new spiritual reality and changed her view of Christians forever. She was studying at the Catholic college forty miles from her hometown. Because she was older and more serious than the girls in the undergraduate dormitory, Lily was given a room in the same building as the nuns and an older religious lay-leader, Betty. Though Lily was not Catholic, she found herself adopted, embraced by the religious community—made an integral part of meals, leisure activities, buzz sessions, and Bible studies. Even though Lily could not partake of the Sacrament, or "Communion" as she called it, she went with the nuns daily to mass and felt the same consolation and warmth as she had experienced previously in the quiet ritual of traditional Episcopalian services. Lily was almost happy.

One balmy autumn evening, early in her first semester, Lily slid open her dorm room window and listened to joyous singing that floated up from the chapel below. She had just caught the words, "They'll know we are Christians by our love", when unexpectedly there was a knock on her dorm room door, and a young nun bounced in excitedly. "Well, don't just sit there. Come on. We are redecorating the chapel, and we need your help."

"But---but I'm not Catholic."

"So? You're Christian," insisted the Sister, her brown and white habit bobbing as she talked. "Come on."

As Lily helped move furniture, hang banners, and arrange flowers, Betty approached her, her usual smile wavering. "Lily, we're so glad you are with us. But I have to tell you about a big disappointment I had today."

Oh, dear, what did I do now? Lily wondered.

"Remember when you told Father you missed being able to take the Blessed Sacrament, like you had in the Episcopal Church? He asked his superior if, in light of the growing ecumenicalism, you might take the Sacrament here at the college. Today his superior told Father that he could not grant that permission. I'm sorry. I hope you will continue to celebrate mass with us."

Lily stood stunned. She had mentioned the Eucharist only in passing and did not expect to be allowed to participate. Even in her parents' church, she was not welcome at Communion. Why should these strangers exert themselves for her? She wanted to tell them all how much their love and acceptance meant to her, but the words came out stilted.

"Thank you for asking, Betty, and thank Father for me. That's more love than my parents' church ever showed me. I can still enjoy mass because I'm worshiping with Christians who want me."

Lily dived into physical work to escape further conversation. When no one would miss her, she slipped out into the starlit night. A cool breeze fluttered the falling maple leaves. Over the lake, the moon dipped low in greeting. Softly, Lily whispered. "Jesus, it was said of You, 'He came unto His own and His own received Him not.' 'I was a stranger and you took me in.' I understand how You felt. I told You years ago that I wanted identification with You. But I thought of 'Identification with Christ' as some high, sanctimonious thing. Instead, following in Your steps means understanding Your feelings, including pain, rejection, and humiliation. I thank you even for my rejection from my parents' church, because that is what You experienced at Nazareth.

"And thank you also for these strangers who made me a part of their family. I ask a special blessing for Betty, and Father, and the Sisters who love You. You said, 'In as much as you have done it unto the least of these, you have done it unto Me.' What they have done for me, they have done for You. Remember them, Jesus."

As Lily slid into bed later that night, she observed aloud, "Jesus, forgiveness is expensive, isn't it? It cost You Your life when You bore the brunt of Your anger at our sins instead of letting us have what we deserve." Lily stared at the wooden crucifix on the wall next to her bed. "But once the cross was over, it was over. You continually let go of the hurt we give You and don't hold us responsible anymore. You have to be unimaginably strong to do that. I've always wanted to forgive like You do, but I couldn't. I just didn't have the ego-strength to handle my reactions to hurt. Being accepted and loved tonight has allowed me to appreciate what has happened to me and has made me strong enough to take the responsibility for my own feelings. Now I can forgive. Thank you for giving me the power to forgive the hurtful teachers, and preachers, and all those others. Good night."

That evening, and the nuns' continual acceptance, gave Lily courage to try visiting a church of her parents' denomination. She had avoided all similar churches since being rejected from her parents' congregation. One snowy Sunday morning in December, Lily wrapped that courage around herself like a blanket and drove to a large church near the college. Keeping her head down, she crept inside, trying not to be noticed. As she hung up her grey wool coat on a rack in the hall, she watched a dozen young women standing together, talking and laughing. To her dismay, one of them turned, looked straight at her, and walked in her direction. Panicked, Lily glanced around for an escape, but there was no place to hide.

"Hello!" the young woman in a chic brown pantsuit called cheerily. "Don't I know you from somewhere?" Before Lily could reply, the woman reached out to shake hands. "I know. You were in my classroom videotaping last week. You are from the special education department." Lily smiled weakly and nodded. "I'm sorry, I forgot your name."

"I'm Lily Farmer. I enjoyed watching you teach those little deaf children. You're Barb, uh...."

"Barb Matins. But call me Babs. Come on, Lily. I'll introduce you to our bunch. We're all pretty chummy here."

To Lily's shock and delight, she found herself pulled into the group of young professionals. Before the morning was over, she was invited to their mid-week Bible study and to a Christmas party at Babs' home. Lily had found friends and a church that would be her own for the remainder of her years in the city.

January 1972

The fourth incident centered on a brief conversation Lily had with her major professor during her second year of graduate study at the Catholic college. As Lily tidied up the special education library one morning, her major professor strolled in. A comfortably rounded middle-aged man with a laughing voice, he had always encouraged Lily to be relaxed with him, and that had brought out the best of Lily's abilities.

"What are you doing here so early?" Lily quipped from behind a table covered in file folders.

"I wanted to catch you before you had books piled around your ears and wouldn't hear me. We need to work out a couple of things. Can you man the resource center every other Saturday so we can keep it open for teachers from out of the area?"

Lily hesitated. She saw her psychiatrist in the state capitol every Saturday but she had never mentioned him to her major professor. "I—I usually have a doctor's appointment on Saturday, but if you need me--."

"Yes, I know you had some trouble when you first started college here but I think you can miss some appointments now. Don't you?"

Lily calculated quickly, and then grinned in self-satisfaction. "Sure, I can do it."

"Good, I'll give you the keys so you can open up. Also, a student with cerebral palsy is coming to work here as an assistant. I want you to set up a program for her. Train her in skills she can use on future jobs. Also, we will have several undergraduate work-study students coming in. Teach them to take over the routine library tasks. I want to free you to do research for me that needs your expertise."

Lily beamed. "Fine, but don't let those undergrads mess up my filing system," Lily quipped laughingly, pointing to the piles on the table. As the professor disappeared from the room, Lily mused, *so he knew all along. My roommate must have told him. But he never treated me like anything was wrong with me. So I never acted like anything was wrong. As Prof Filbert used to say, 'Unconditional acceptance with positive regard leads to' ...hmmm...I'd say, leads to success."*

April—May 1972

Just before Lily graduated with her master's degree, she dropped psychiatric therapy. Outwardly she appeared well adjusted. But inwardly she felt her psychiatrist had nothing more to teach her. He had been kind, considerate, and wise, but he could not help with the immediate difficulty disrupting Lily's daily life, what she called a *lack of emotional glue.*

I just come unglued, she thought. *I have no definite shape or design. I'm like a complex mosaic whose glue dries out and whose pieces fall all over the floor.*

Instinctively, Lily sensed that the *glue* lay somewhere in the integration of her Christian beliefs with her daily life. But even though her psychiatrist was a Christian, he regarded Lily's myriad of spiritual questions as merely theoretical and theological and avoided discussing them.

Neither was popular Christian literature any help to Lily. After reading one well-known book, she commented to herself, "The difference between their emotional problems and mine is the difference between a scab and a cancer. They are solving problems I'm not even well enough to have."

On the day that she graduated with her master's degree, Lily wrote in her journal:
"Take finger paint. Create millions of intricate, finely colored figures. Make each slightly different and yet an integral part of the painting. Put your finger on one shape and rub it into colorless, formless oblivion. The result is naquan. I am naquan.

>The world is sad.
>The mask is glad.
>Without the mask
>>Life is bad.
>And they tell us to be ourselves?"

CHAPTER 19—THE CRASH
March 1974—2 years later

Lily Farmer screamed, throwing herself frantically onto her bed. Light crashed against light, breaking into sharp prisms of red and blue, dancing menacingly toward her face. Intense rays of sunlight cut jagged patterns on the bedroom windowpane, threatening to shatter it into a thousand razor-edged fragments.

Lily buried her head under the pillow. Her body curled into a tense fetal ball as if to protect her vital parts from the merciless light, from the mental aberration that looked so real. The pillow blocked out the light, but it could not block the splintering and crackling in her head. "No! No!" Lily screamed again. "Go away! Go away! Oh, God, I can't stand it."

The cry released part of the inner pain, and with the release, the hallucination subsided. Lily held herself rigidly still. She knew she must get help; she must not stay alone lest the hallucination return and overpower her. No one else was in the house; the lady with whom she boarded was away for the day. Gradually Lily convinced herself to open her eyes. The bedroom walls and windows still swayed and the sharp light hurt her eyes. But the floor was stable and the nameless fear lessening. Braving the remaining distortions, Lily stumbled to the telephone in the dining room and dialed the number of a friend who headed the inner city counseling ministry where she often volunteered.

"Warren, Warren, I'm sorry to bother you at home, but I'm cracking up again. Please, I have to see you…. Yes, I think I can drive. Thank you, I'll be there in twenty minutes."

Glassy-eyed, Lily drove across the city, slowly,

deliberately, hoping that her vision would steer her through the real world without collision.

Soon she was seated in Warren's well-worn living room, facing her trusted friend. Warren, bearded with long hair and blue jeans, was a highly skilled counselor who did not bother with professional trappings. In his comfortable presence, Lily stopped struggling to maintain sight and hearing: she let the fog settle in, muffling the sharp sounds, and softening the painful light.

"Warren, I lost my job." Through the fog, Lily searched Warren's face for signs of disapproval. Finding only love, she continued, "I only have five weeks more to work. I can't take it, not one more time. I tried to do my work well, but the hospital unit director said I just didn't fit. Warren, I'm different! I never fit!"

"I didn't think you liked the job anyway, Lily."

"Working in an institution with untoilet-trained retarded adults? Who would?" Lily sniffed. " But the job is over each day at 4:00 and it pays good money. I need the money to be free. Now I'll never be able to get another job."

Warren stretched out his long legs and laced his hands behind his head, acting as if there were no problem at all. "Lily, there will be other jobs. When you lost the job in the lab six years ago, you thought that was the end. Was it?"

"No."

"No, since then you have had three jobs where your bosses liked you."

"They were just temporary jobs."

"Then last year when you were asked to resign from teaching school, you thought you would never find a job, but you did and in the same city where you went to grad school so you didn't have to leave your church and friends. In less than a month, you had a job with more prestige, more money, and less work. You're well educated in three separate areas; you will find another job."

"No, Warren, no. Not this time. I can't take it. I

can't face the world. I'm cracking up. I'm losing everything." Head down, Lily wrapped her arms around herself protectively.

"All right. So what is the worst thing that can happen to you now?"

"To end up in the psychiatric ward again," she mumbled.

"Is that so bad? You have done it before," he asked in a nonchalant tone.

Before Lily's eyes flashed ancient pictures: Lily shrieking at her wide-eyed, innocent college roommate; an elderly dean of women, face contorting in condemnation; fire and breaking glass; a troll-like doctor rejecting her. But, finally, from the mist, a glob of red took form, red hair on a stately head—the red-haired psychiatrist who had liked Lily and given her blessed protection in the hospital ward.

"No," Lily admitted to Warren, "the hospital was not so bad, less scary than the outside world." She looked up toward her friend.

"So the hospital is the worst, and now you have faced that." Warren's face was serious, but his voice was grinning. "You have had lots of upsets and near breaks in the last six years, but you have learned from each one and grown stronger. So if you fall apart and have to go to a hospital now, go! Have a good rest. You are a fighter by nature and you will come out stronger again."

"I suppose so," Lily said, sounding unconvinced, though Warren's matter-of-fact attitude had made the real world seem more survivable.

Warren reached for a pad of paper and wrote down a name and phone number. "Lily, before you give up, I want you to see a Christian psychiatrist who is new in town. He can give you more help than I can. I'll even call and make the appointment."

"No thanks," she replied, taking the note. "I can do that much for myself. He is probably another dead end, but if you want me to, I'll see him."

CHAPTER 20—FIRST ENCOUNTER
March 1974

Five days after her promise to Warren, Lily strode across the court of an elegant office mall with her head erect, smiling mask in place, trying to look as if she were not going to see a psychiatrist. The high heel of her left dress boot caught in the carpet. "Darn leg thinks it can do as it pleases, always reminding me I'm not like those women," she grumbled softly, glaring at the graceful, efficient secretaries flowing between offices, flawless in their presentation.

Lily found the door marked "Louis E. Best, M.D." and marched in, hiding behind a façade of disinterest. She took the clipboard full of paperwork that the secretary handed her and seated herself in a small, private waiting area. With brutal honesty, she filled out the detailed questionnaire about her history and present life. Then she leaned back in the wooden straight chair and watched the white rain dropping from the ceiling. She doubted that this psychiatrist was anything more special than an additional link in the long chain of therapists. But, for the sake of the possibility, she would endure the interview.

A tall, well-built man with a square face and broad smile, in his 40's, approached her. "You're Lily Farmer? I'm Dr. Best. I'm glad to meet you. Let's go back to my office."

Lily followed the doctor and seated herself in a metal folding chair that faced a window overlooking a green lawn. The office was bare, except for the four folding chairs and a worn bookcase, and, in a gold frame behind the desk, the classic Sallman's Head of Christ.

Dr. Best pulled a chair up at an angle to Lily's and sat down as relaxed as if they were old friends getting together for a social visit, and commented, " My office furniture hasn't arrived yet. I have only been in town for three weeks."

Taking the clipboard from Lily, Dr. Best read through the questionnaire, making comments and inquiries. "You have quite a record of accomplishments. Counselor in a correctional institution, teacher of the retarded, psychological assistant in a state hospital. Christian. You know Jesus as your Friend."

As he paused and looked up at Lily, she felt the world start to spin. What would a psychiatrist say about that statement? To her surprise, he commented casually, "Good. So do I," and returned to the form. For Lily, the world steadied again. Dr. Best continued looking at her answers. "Immediate problem—losing your job because you could not get along with the staff." He laid aside the clipboard and said, "Tell me about your relationships on the job."

Lily described in bald, unflattering terms her confusion about her duties, her constant misinterpretations of her bosses and fellow employees, and her inability to make friends at work.

Without comment, Dr. Best turned back to the questionnaire. "Hmm. Long term problem—recurrence of former schizophrenia." Now the psychiatrist surveyed Lily keenly. "What do you mean by *schizophrenia?* That term doesn't mean much to me."

"I live in detachment; the world is a picture and I must constantly step into it, hoping it won't move around and fall. I see colors, lights, sometimes objects that I know can't be there. More often, my vision is cut off, like there is a fog before my eyes. My feeling and thinking won't work together. I think about beauty and automatically hate it. I try to be nice and good, but end up hostile. Dr. Best, I have been in and out of therapy for eight years, ever since my sophomore year in college. I thought I had my lesser self under control, but I know the signs, and I am about to crack up. It's disgusting and infuriating, and I don't understand why I can't help myself."

"You are saying that you don't understand what happens to you periodically. You have difficulty understanding roles and what people expect of you and how to react in social situations. And there is no one else in your life now who understands you." Dr. Best raised his bushy eyebrows questioningly. "Have you heard of learning disabilities?"

"Yes! Yes!" Lily answered enthusiastically at the mention of an area of her academic expertise. "My special education training included diagnosing learning disabilities in reading. I've been toying with the similarities in perceptual problems of children with learning disabilities and the distortions of adults with schizophrenia." Abruptly, she became aware of her own verbosity. "Oh, excuse my rambling. Why are you asking?"

"One kind of learning disability is an inability to understand social roles. Your job problem sounds as if you constantly collide with social roles that you misperceive."

They discussed roles and jobs for a few minutes. Feeling comfortable with this man, Lily decided to risk more honesty than she usually bestowed so early in a relationship. His response to this test would indicate whether she could trust Dr. Best with even more devastating confidences.

"Dr. Best, all that is fine, but it doesn't explain the hate, the inner violence, the physical symptoms. And if I'm not schizophrenic, then I'm illegitimate. Then all these problems aren't real. I have to hear and see and have energy and function like everyone else. But I can't."

"If you are not schizophrenic, then you are lazy and worthless and making up the whole thing?" Dr. Best smiled gently.

"Yes, that is why I was so relieved when my college professor told me that I was schizophrenic." Lily stopped. "Wait a minute. How did you know that? None of my therapists understood that."

"I have seen too many parents and teachers imply that a child is lazy and no-good.
A label to you means a right to be what you are. In this office you may be, hear, see, or think whatever you like. You don't need a label, and you don't have to live up to any image. You can be yourself."

"That's a lousy thing to be," Lily retorted. Then, to cover up her self-exposure, she added, "What about the symptoms?"

"Perceptual disorders may be caused by brain malfunction. Have you had an EEG?"

"Three of them. They don't show a thing."

"Well, medical science still has a lot to learn about measuring brain functioning. Someday in the future, when our technology improves, you may want to pursue further neurological evaluation. But for now, you know what you experience. Accept your experience as valid. You don't have to explain everything that happens, not even to yourself."

Plus one for you. Lily mentally scored her test of Dr. Best with an A plus. Now she dared risk deeper emotional involvement. She stared out the window for a minute, and then looked at a spot on the wall slightly to the right of the psychiatrist.

"Dr. Best, what about all the hate and guilt and fear? I don't want them. I want—I want love and peace and joy. But conventional Christian formulas haven't worked and have left me feeling more hurt and alone. Recently the pressure inside me is mounting to the point I'm afraid I'll explode and do something dumb like I did years ago."

"Maybe you are caught in a cycle." Lily frowned at him questioningly. " Peter's writing as translated in the Amplified Version of the Bible may give us a clue." Dr. Best pulled a worn red Bible from his shelf and said, "This is from II Peter chapter 1. 'May grace (God's favor) and peace (which is perfect well-being, all necessary good…freedom from fears and agitating passions…) be multiplied to you in (the full, personal, precise and correct) knowledge of God....' Our peace is founded on a full and correct knowledge of God. If our knowledge is incorrect, then our feelings will be distorted, and our actions, immature or inappropriate."

"I don't understand what you mean by a cycle," Lily interrupted.

"The cycle goes like this. First, we think—including what we have learned and stored in our unconscious reservoir of experiences. Second, based on what we think, we feel. Third, based on our thinking and feeling, we act. The actions tend to validate what we originally thought."

"Thinking, feeling, then action." Lily ticked the three off on her fingers. " Now apply that to God, please."

"If we picture God the Father as a tyrant, we feel afraid. If we think of Him as unpredictable, we feel insecure. We act on the fear or insecurity, and the unsatisfactory results of the actions tend to confirm our fear and insecurity. But if we know the Father's unconditional acceptance of us in Christ, we experience peace, security, and confidence. Perhaps you need to know this acceptance."

"Peter wrote about psychology like that?" Lily felt a faint thrill. Dr. Best was using the Bible, the book that had been used to condemn her, as a source of hope. Could he possibly have real answers? From self-protective habit, however, she pushed away the hope and continued to intellectualize. "I like the idea of thinking first. Learning can change thinking and I know how to learn. But I don't understand the relationship of this to my hang-ups with guilt and the inability to feel love."

Sensing Lily's bewilderment about unconditional acceptance, Dr. Best changed his approach. "You have been telling me that you are afraid, afraid of your own impulses. You have also been showing me that you measure yourself against a standard of total selfless love. Perhaps you expect more of yourself than is realistic at this point in your development. Have you heard of the spiral of spiritual maturity?"

"No. Sounds interesting."

Dr. Best picked up the Bible again and flipped to a book-marked passage. "The characteristics of maturity develop in a sequential order, one step at a time, and we relive the cycle repeatedly on higher and higher levels. If you read II Peter 1:5-7 in the Amplified Version, you see that for Christ's nature to fully develop in us, we must diligently practice acting on the divine promises. First comes faith. Then exercising faith will develop virtue, or excellence."

Lily stifled a giggle. The word *exercising* had conjured up a picture of a gym-like room with a sign "Practice Divine Promises Here." She saw herself doing a set of energetic calisthenics called *faith-ercises*, which resulted in excellence, with her feeling tall and strong. However, Lily was not about to share her humorous picture with this psychiatrist so earnestly trying to help her. She forced her attention back to what Dr. Best was saying.

"Exercising virtue develops knowledge. Exercising knowledge develops self-control, which includes confidence that we can express feelings appropriately."

"I thought self-control was NOT doing things," Lily muttered.

Dr. Best smiled and continued. "After self-control comes patience with self and others. Then godliness. Then brotherly love. And finally, the love by which you have measured yourself, agape love, loving others selflessly as God love us."

"No wonder I'm frustrated!" Lily said. "I understand about knowledge. But I don't trust my self-control, and I'm expecting myself to perform four stages later in the sequence. You are saying that I don't need to expect so much from myself." Dr. Best nodded. Lily let out a long breath. "What a relief!"

"Your inadequate self-expression may be based on faulty knowledge of yourself, the world, or God."

"Oh, so we begin again with knowledge. That I can

deal with."

"Yes, with knowledge. But I'm sorry; our time is up. If you want to see me for therapy, we will explore who you are in your eyes and in God's. Do you want to plan therapy sessions each week?"

"I think I had better. You make sense." Lily could not allow herself a simple *yes*, which would imply that she was entitled to what she wanted, something that Lily was not yet ready to believe.

Guarding firmly against the exhilaration threatening to break through the intellectual façade, Lily hurried through the formalities of leaving the office. Once outside the building, however, she bounded across the parking lot, jumped into her red Chevy, and burst out, "God, thank You. Thank You for Dr. Best. He has answers, real answers. He has a plan; he doesn't just wander like most therapists. He understands me. He doesn't condemn with IAYH—it's all in your head—when I talk about the physical symptoms. And he knows You. Maybe there is hope."

CHAPTER 21—WORLDS IN COLLISION
March 1974

The evening following her first encounter with Dr. Best, Lily lay stretched out on her bed, hands behind her head, alone in her comfortable room in Lena' s house where she had boarded for the past two years since graduating from the Catholic college. Absently, she watched the shadows dancing on the ceiling, shadows of tree branches waving before the streetlight that shone through the wide window at the head of her bed. She had put on her red fleece pajamas early but was not in the least sleepy. The session with Dr. Best filled her mind. Her original enthusiasm about the session was dying out, as frustration and confusing accusations from her unconscious forced themselves into her awareness.

"I wish Lena were here so I could talk out some of this," she said to herself. The imminently practical, middle-aged Lena was away at a Bible study for the evening. "But then, maybe I shouldn't tell Lena about Dr. Best. She is so healthy-minded that she probably couldn't understand seeing a psychiatrist."

Searching for a sounding board for the conflict churning within her, Lily sat up, turned on the crystal lamp on her bedside table, and pulled her green journal and pen out of its drawer. Letting her subconscious mind take over, she wrote rapidly.

"The world is a cold and hostile thing,
Little joy and peace it brings,
Yet somehow I cannot bear,
Not to love life and call it fair."

Sucking on the end of her Lindy ballpoint pen, she re-read the verse, then began writing more slowly and deliberately. "Dr. Best stirs up hope that life can improve.

But I have hoped and been crushed so often; surely I know better than to hope again. Yet, no one has ever talked to me like Dr. Best has. He applied the Bible so that it is friendly, instead of condemning. He listened and seemed to genuinely care about me—like I am a special person instead of just a patient. He didn't discount the turbulence of my feelings, forcing me to hysterics to prove them.

"But Dr. Best's acceptance and skill also make him dangerous. He has the power to lure me into trusting him with too many secrets. Even today, our first meeting, I trusted him. If I tell him more, can he protect me against the punishment I will receive from my own mind for revealing its hidden parts? Can the doctor himself be trusted? Or will he force from me the truth and then wield it as a sword to destroy me? I fear."

With her journal open on her lap, Lily reached for her worn Bible, intending to find the passage in Ephesians 6 about the Christian's spiritual armor to protect her from that fear. But instead, as she opened the book, her eyes fixed on the chapter's first three verses. "Children, obey your parents in the Lord: for this is right. Honor thy father and mother…That it may be well with thee, and thou mayest live long on the earth."

To Lily's disturbed mind, these verses leaped out at her, mocking, taunting her. She grabbed up her pen and scrawled, "Why, God? Why do You not keep your promises? Or am I so different that the promises don't apply to me?

"I did obey my parents—to the last letter of the law and beyond, even trying to guess what they would want next, and doing that too. I spent the first eighteen years of my life trying to take care of them and make them happy. So, if the Bible is true, why is it not well with me? Or do the promises not apply to me? Maybe I really am not human."

A dense fog of despair settled around Lily's head. "Perhaps I do not belong in this world," she droned, lying down and curling into a ball. "I should leave."

As quick as the utterance, Lily's mind left the time/space world for the world of madness. All night she knew only outer darkness with grotesque shapes and terrifying beasts sailing through it, mocking and ridiculing her. Several times she saw herself once again standing at the mouth of a black rubber tunnel floating in darkness. Behind her, the conduit's yawning throat threatened to engulf her if she stepped backwards. Before her stretched only the vast emptiness of space. She stood still, afraid to move, bracing herself with her hands against the sides of the tunnel. All night she endured the terrors of imagination untouched by reason.

Miraculously, the first soft rays of morning light pouring through her window penetrated the nightmare world, drawing Lily gently back to Earth. She opened her eyes and was relieved to find her room in its usual orderly array. Lily Farmer shook herself the rest of the way into reality, then looked at her calendar clock.

"Wednesday, March 27, 1974," she muttered. "Another day on the nasty job. Oh, well, even my job beats the tunnel. I haven't been in that tunnel since I left the psych ward six years ago. I hope it doesn't mean I'm going to be that sick again. Ish!"

Promptly at 8:00 a.m. that morning, Lily unlocked, entered, and re-locked the double doors of the brick building housing the severely retarded residents at the state hospital. Crossing the grim lobby, she unlocked the metal door of the nurses' station and signed in on the time sheet marked "Professional Staff." "Professional," she grumbled under her breath. "The only thing professional about our psychology staff is that we *profess* to have authority. These crude, uneducated attendants are the ones who really run this unit. What I wouldn't give for the power to fire every one of them and bring in people who would love these kids."

As she shoved the time sheet into the proper drawer, Lily heard the attendant supervisor bellowing from the doorway that opened into the residents' hall.

"Hey, you! Yeah, you!"

Lily turned around.

"We got no attendant down on Ward B. That therapy kid, that nasty Stevie of yours, is down there. Go keep him company—and mind the rest of the brats while you're at it."

More cleaning up crud, Lily thought. *Not quite what I was hired to do.* She looked down at her neat red pants suit and ruffled blouse and sighed. But without a word she obligingly trudged down the concrete and tile hall to Ward B.

Lily opened the ward door, and then slammed it, grabbing her stomach, trying not to heave. Apparently the ward had been without an attendant overnight. Human excrement covered the gray tile floor. One girl was playing in the toilets. Several children were stark naked. The boy with Down's syndrome was bruised and bleeding where he beat his head against the wall. And Stevie, her therapy case, was still tied to the bed, hands tightly bound together against his chest, gown soaked in urine. Praying for courage, Lily waded into the blood and gore. By the time Ward B was called to breakfast, the floor was mopped and the children were clean and dressed.

Lily had taken extra time with Stevie. First she had broken the string made of rags that fastened him to the bed. Tying wandering residents to their beds was an illegal, but common, practice. Then Lily unbound the child's hands and stroked his tousled brown hair. Gently she rubbed circulation into the bony limbs, crooning to him, "Stevie, Stevie, he's my bo-ey. He's a good boy." The hand tying had begun as a therapeutic procedure to stop Stevie from beating his face with his fist and to allow the open red sore on his cheek to heal. But though the cheek was improved, attendants continued to tie the boy's hands.

Lily let Stevie stand in the shower as long as he liked, then gave him clean clothes. Stevie slid himself into the institutional gray denim trousers and pullover shirt. "Stevie, I think you learned to beat your face because you were bored and wanted some kind of stimulation, like a baby seeking touch and motion. Let's try you in the play therapy room this afternoon."

When the afternoon shift arrived, Lily was free to take Stevie to her therapeutic playroom equipped with blocks, a small wagon, a sand box, and other toys appropriate for children with a mental age of two. Though Stevie was seventeen years old, his mind was that of a toddler and his body less than four feet tall. Lily coaxed her patient. "Come on, Stevie. Let's play in the sand box. Put your hand in. See how good the sand feels. That's it, Stevie! What the—."

Stevie had stooped down and stirred his fingers through the grains of sand, then jumped back wailing in fright. Impulsively, Lily wrapped her arms around the child and immediately the howling dwindled to sniffles.

"Is Stevie scared? Does he need a mommy?" Lily spied the rocking chair in the corner and pulled him over to it. "Come on, Stevie. Be my baby."

Lily gathered the child's slim frame onto her lap and rocked. Stevie nestled his head against her shoulder. The mucus from his perpetually runny nose stained Lily's snow-white blouse, but she did not care. She had found a way to reach a child previously considered impossible.

"Oh, Stevie, you just want to be a baby and have a mommy. You've lived in this old institution most of your life, and no one cares. I wonder if I can give you enough security and love before I leave here so that you stop beating your face. Maybe we can even prove that you can participate in play activities: then you can go to class and have something else to do with those hands. Poor little hands."

Lily rubbed the claw-like fingers. From lack of use, Stevie's fingers and arms were stiff and permanently crooked. "I bet no one ever tried to exercise those little arms to see if they would move." Lily began singing "Ten Little Indians" while bending Stevie's right arm back and forth at the elbow in time with the music. She heard a funny gurgle next to her shoulder. Then a red little face turned up to greet her—a red face with a big smile.

"Stevie, you smiled!" Lily sang for joy, "Stevie, Stevie, Stevie smiled...." To her knowledge, no one had ever seen the boy smile.

When therapy ended, Lily led Stevie, hands unbound, back to his ward, singing to him. As she walked him through the ward door, the attendant growled, "The face-banger's back. Here, brat, have a string and tie yourself. Or better yet, hang yourself."

Lily grabbed the rag string. "Stevie is not to be tied. Treat him gently and he will stop hitting himself."

Lily stopped by the nurses' station and quickly wrote a treatment plan for gentle care, mothering, and no restraints. But even as she wrote, she knew the futility of her plan. These attendants were rough with their own children; why would they be gentle with retarded people? Hoping to find an ally among the attendant staff, Lily sought out an elderly black lady who sometimes worked on Ward B. Finding her writing at the desk in the staff records room, Lily asked, "Did you ever see little Stevie on Ward B smile?"

"No, don't believe I have. I sure would like to see something done for that tyke."

"Well, today Stevie smiled." Lily related the story and then pleaded, "Could you talk to the other attendants about helping Stevie? I'm white and professional staff: they won't listen to me, but they might to you."

"I don't know. I'm not well liked. Not even by the boss lady up front. She says I spoil the kids. But then, you ought to hear what she says about you."

"I can guess. Will you at least try to talk to the others?"

"I'll try. I sure wish I could be down there with those young ones all the time. Might be able to help them. I asked once; I'll never ask again."

"I understand," Lily murmured. "Thanks for whatever you can do."

Still elated over her success, Lily hurried to get her belongings from her office and signed out at the nurses' station. Once she was outdoors, an episode of uncontrollable enthusiasm caught her, sending Lily skipping and hopping across the parking lot like a seven-year-old at a birthday party. As she started the engine of her red Chevy, Lily repeated excitedly, "I did it. I did it. I did it."

"Lena, I did it!" Lily bubbled as she burst through the front door of her home.

Lena's red hair and freckled face appeared over the top of the newspaper she was reading at the shiny Formica-topped dining table. "You did what? Flew without wings?'

"I made Stevie smile."

"Slow down, honey. Is Stevie one of your kids? Come down to earth and tell me what happened."

Seating herself across from Lena, Lily told about taking Stevie to the playroom, about his cuddling against her as she rocked him, and about the big smile on his tear-streaked face.

"Lily, you really love those kids, don't you? I couldn't do that job. The time you brought one of the better girls home was too much for me."

"I do love them. I guess I understand them. They just want to be accepted for who they are and treated with kindness and decency. Can you imagine what would happen if seventy two-year-old normal children were placed in a big room and made to sit in chairs and do nothing all day? That's what we do with those residents of two-year-old mentality—and then wonder why they behave so badly."

"Lily, when you put yourself into the work the way you do, I can't see why you were fired."

"I don't fit, Lena. I don't fit in with the rest of the staff. According to the unit director, I upset the program— what program I don't know. I disrupt staff morale. I bring in too many new ideas. It's the same old story I have heard all my life. I just don't belong. I'm different."

"You belong here, Lily. I can't see anything so different about you. My daughter looks up to you. You're like part of the family."

"But, Lena, I get along here because of your attitude. You accept me just as I am. You don't demand that I be 'big and bad' like the attendants. Or 'happy all the time' like my former church expected. Or brilliant and successful. You give me permission to be myself."

"Are you different at work than you are here?"

"I probably am. I try to mind my own business and speak politely. But I hate those attendants for their filthy, loud mouths and their cruelty. And I imagine that hate shows through."

"Do you really hate them?"

"Yes, I do. I don't want to. I pray to love them. But every time I go into that building and live with their vileness, I hate them."

"Well, you won't have to be around them much longer." Lena folded the newspaper and laid it on the floor beside the tubular steel leg of her chair. "Say, I didn't get to see you yesterday. Did you go to that new doctor?"

"Yes. His name is Dr. Best."

"How do you like him?" Lena asked as she went to the stove to start supper.

"He scares me, but I like him. Or maybe I'm scared because I like him, and people I like have power to hurt."

"What did you say, Lily?" Lena asked, picking up a pan that had clattered to the floor. "I didn't hear all that."

"Oh, never mind." Lily was disgusted at herself for saying so much. "I like Dr. Best. He may even be able to help me."

"Fine. Would you mind cutting up some salad?"

Lily chuckled at Lena's trick of turning to practical work whenever the conversation bordered on the emotional.

*****

Sunday night after church, Lily slouched on her bed, her back against the maple headboard, her pillow and journal on her lap, trying to prepare herself for the next week of work. In her journal, she wrote: "Rejected, but expected to show up and work. Not worth having around, but superwoman, expected to do what no one else can. Life is always like that. I wish I could escape.

"I could. There is one place where I am wanted and competent—the Island." As quickly as that, she shifted into her Shawn frame-of-reference. "I have been sticking to my intelligence work in America and letting the islanders come to me for the past two years. I thought maybe the last psychiatrist might be right, that I couldn't handle both worlds. But maybe, just maybe–" She dropped her pen and grumbled, "Oh, fiddle, I don't know." Petulantly, she picked up a current events magazine. "Wonder if there is anything in here that affects the Island."

A photograph of Buddhist priests in political protest glared back at her from the magazine. The article read, "Saffron-robed priests swirled about the campfire, their chants echoing through the Indian night, summoning youths to their cause. Shrill music mingled with the eerie night sounds as–"

Pain and explosive pressure swept through Lily. "No! No! I can't allow this. I have to go back to the Island."

Lost to the time/space existence, Lily was hurled back into her fantasy kingdom. She felt the flying pack on her back lift her into the sky and felt the mighty rush of wind through her hair. Far below her, she glimpsed the churning blue of the ocean, a string of jade green islands, then just one island with a lone palm protruding from the low, sandy beach. She cried to the wind, "Lily, stay behind. Shawn forever be Shawn of Lone Palm Island, fearless, forceful, free."

As in dreams, scenes swam before her eyes, and then vanished. She was standing on the beach in the center of a thatched village. A tan-skinned multitude in oriental dress surged about her, shouting in a foreign language, "The Queen is come. Our Shawn is come home." A white silk robe with a tiger embroidered in gold settled over her pale shoulders. Then she was sitting on a high throne of black stone, the crowd bowing around her. Before her glided saffron-robed figures, the rebel priests, chanting, "Beware, beware, you have been telling secrets, beware."

The scene changed. She was lying on a richly draped bed, with hangings of green and gold and blue, idly stroking the head of a great Bengal tiger, her pet and protector. The tiger rested his huge velvet paw on her shoulder as if trying to comfort her. "It's all right, Tiger," she whispered, reassuring herself as much as her pet. "I have fought for my throne before, and the false priest accusers have never won. Watch over me tonight and tomorrow I shall fight again."

The mind of Shawn lay down to sleep; the body of Lily in the blue and green room at Lena's pulled the plaid blankets over her head and, arm around her stuffed toy tiger, slept.

The next morning, at the demand of the alarm clock, the body of Lily and the mind of Shawn united to assault another earthly Monday. As she dressed in a tailored dark pants and tunic, she remarked to no one in particular, "If Monday must come, at least it is I, Shawn, the competent one, who faces it—not her Lily-liveredness."

Forty-five minutes later, the pseudo-ego Shawn strode aggressively into the cafeteria of the unit for severely retarded. She would not cower before the vulgarity of the lower class; she would be in charge. She surveyed the dining hall and immediately her eyes fixed on the line of residents waiting for breakfast trays. At the rear of the line, blood running down his face, stood Stevie howling. A large gash lay open on the top of his head. His hands were tied against his chest.

"Why are Stevie's hands tied? What happened to his head?" She demanded answers of the attendant standing indolently beside the line.

"Don't ask me. He come down here that a-way."

"Who is on duty on his ward?"

"Don't know. Simmons is on medication and treatment."

Hugging the child, the psychologist untied his hands. "Come on, Stevie, let's get your head cleaned up." Her arm around his shoulders, she guided the boy toward the treatment room.

As she left the cafeteria, one of the few male patients who could speak tugged at her tunic. "Miss Lily, Jamison done it. Pushed him into the bed rail. His hands was tied. Couldn't help hisself."

Lily laid a gentle hand of appreciation on the man's shoulder. "Thanks, friend."

In the treatment room, Simmons roughly disinfected and bandaged Stevie's cut. "Do you know who was on duty on Ward B this morning?" Lily hoped that at least this practical nurse would be her ally in protecting the children.

"I don't know nothing and don't want to. You educated people baby these brats too much."

Lily sighed and put her arm around the boy's shoulder. As she guided him back to the cafeteria line, the child snuggled against her. "It's okay, Stevie. I love you."

At the serving hatch, Lily met with more hostility from the cook who grumbled that "retards" who were late deserved to miss breakfast. But seeing the fire of vengeance smoldering in the psychologist's eyes, the cook slammed a tray of cold food on the counter and walked away. Lily led Stevie to an empty table and stayed with him until he finished eating, to insure that the food would not be snatched away by a hurried attendant.

After taking Stevie to his ward, Lily retreated to her office. Muttering, she rummaged on her desk for an incident report form. "These so-and-so's hit the kids, tie them up, and starve them. Then they say I don't belong here. Hah!"

Switching to the competent Shawn-self, she found

the form and adroitly recorded the bare facts of Stevie's injury under the heading of "accident". "No point in telling the whole story. Jamison has had two hearings for abuse and gotten off. No one is ever fired for abuse, just for caring too much." Then she wrote five well-ordered patient case reports from two-week old notes. "Too bad that when I'm just Lily again I will hardly recognize these reports. They are good."

For the next two days, the Shawn-identity carried out Lily's daily life, adding bits of conversation with visitors from the Island venturing into her American world. Tuesday evening after work she strolled through her housing addition, enjoying the fresh air. Without warning, she heard a voice in her head calling her. Abruptly, the suburban street was transformed into the sandy village road on the Island. "Sister," she protested arrogantly, "these sudden summons between worlds are so draining. I have toyed with the idea of turning the whole rule of the Island over to you permanently. The difficulty is that, in America, Lily could not survive without the Island retreat and without the Shawn competencies. So sad."

CHAPTER 22—I'M DIFFERENT
April 1974

Wednesday afternoon, Shawn strode into Dr. Best's office for her appointment. *Not long for existence—this man won't tolerate unreality*, she thought.

"Hello, Lily," Dr. Best addressed her as she seated herself in a comfortable sky-blue wing chair with a view out the window. Since her first visit, the stark office had been transformed into a room of blue and brown comfort. As Dr. Best took up his position in a fawn-colored recliner at an angle to Lily, he said, "I'm glad to see you. How are you, Lily?"

"Fine." The name, *Lily,* triggered a clash of identities. Her rigidly erect posture slumped a bit. The sparkle died from her eyes. Her hands gripped the chair arms.

"How has your week been?"

Lily sat silently searching for her frame of reference. *A Lily, a dropping flower. Of the time/space world. American. 28 years old. Disturbed. Sitting in a shrink's office. Wednesday, 2:00 p.m.*

Aloud she said, "Fine. Fine, I guess." Lily was not about to confide her clash of worlds to a psychiatrist. Instead she said, "Dr. Best, I'm different."

"What do you mean?" the psychiatrist asked, somewhat startled by the abrupt announcement.

"I used to think I was not human. I know better now. But I am different. You and most people can see, hear, and think all of the time. With me, vision or hearing can simply quit—or be lost in a fog. Sometimes, my mind quits. I don't know what I've done for hours. In college I had reams of notes I never remembered taking. Time stops.

In high school I wanted to be a professional pianist. But in the middle of a Mozart Sonata, time would stop for a few seconds and my fingers would stumble about on their own. The piece would be ruined. And fear, horrible fear, used to sweep over me. Fear of absolutely nothing."

"What you are describing are symptoms. We talked last week about the possibility of brain dysfunction. Some types of nervous system disorders could cause what you are describing."

"You mean maybe these happenings I've condemned as psychological could be physical?"

"Yes, but there is no absolute way to be certain."

Lily fidgeted. "I have a confession to make. I did my graduate research paper on the biochemistry of schizophrenia. Intellectually, I believe that most serious mental illness has a biological component and that the visible results are partly a personality reaction to a body that can't be trusted. But the frustrating part is that I can't convince my whole self. Without hard medical evidence, I still feel responsible, guilty. The only diagnosis I ever had was by the college psychologist. Every other therapist has left me hanging." Lily stared at the toes of her black pumps. "I am so different that I don't even fit a diagnostic category."

"You need a label to have a right to be and to fit somewhere, if only with the sick? Not in my office!" Dr. Best's voice rang with authority. "You have a right to your own experiences. Accept them, good or bad, as your own."

"You believe me?" Lily stared incredulously at the psychiatrist. In spite of her previous tests of this man, she had expected to hear the familiar "just imagining that" or "trying to get attention" answers.

"Certainly I believe you."

"Wow!" was all she could say.

"Sometimes these symptoms come from a biochemical disorder related to diet," Dr. Best was explaining. "If so, a special diet with nutritional supplements may help significantly. I'll loan you a book to read and think about. But the physical symptoms are only one part of your problem. Psychological and spiritual components are as important or more important for you. Thoughts and feelings can change neurochemistry, just as chemistry can change feeling and behavior."

Picking up his cue to re-direct the discussion toward emotional issues, Lily tested the psychiatrist again. "Dr. Best, I see vivid mental pictures that stay with me for years. Sometimes they are about God. For example, one Sunday during my undergraduate days, the front cover of our church bulletin pictured a lady dressed in her Sunday best reaching down her white-gloved hand to a small child. Mentally, I saw God the Father reaching His hand down to take mine. Only, instead of responding happily like the child in the picture, I slapped His hand—hard."

"You distrust authority, don't you? You must have been hurt and disappointed many times."

"How do you know?" Lily's mouth dropped open in surprise. That perceptiveness—how did he see so much? She tried again. "Anyway, this picture came again. A year ago I was going to sleep when I saw God reaching down His hand. The hand was stronger, more loving, less demanding. I wanted to reach out, but I was afraid. I forced my hand toward His, but just out of His grasp."

"Lily, you were learning to be a little less in awe of God and of authority. Did you have any special relationships then?"

"Yes, Warren, a special friend. You know him, I think." Dr. Best nodded. "He helped me with some spiritual problems, and I helped with a few of his counseling cases."

"A friendly authority. Not many of those in your life, I suspect."

Lily smiled at the doctor's insight, although she was determined subconsciously to prove her unworthiness and thereby shake off his concern.

"Last week, after talking with you, I pictured God's hand grasping mine. This time He was bigger than I, but close, loving, friendly. I let Him close His fingers over my hand. Then a fierce impulse came to pull away and run. Dr. Best, that means I want to run away from God and reality. I'm scared."

Dr. Best thought for a moment, then said, "Alter your picture. You envision your relationship with God as depending on you. Try this. Grasp your right hand around your left wrist, your left hand around your right wrist."

Lily followed his instructions, then said, "That's a lock grip, like is used to pull someone out of a hole."

"One hand is yours, the other God's." He demonstrated. "Let go with your hand. What happens?"

"God still has a firm hold on me. I can't slip and I can't run away."

"That's right. God's relationship to you depends on His love, not yours. Like the Apostle Paul said, even when we were sinners, Christ died for us because of His love. We don't have to be worthy."

"But I can still run from God and reality. I have before."

"Picture Jesus." He paused, waiting until her eye movement showed that she was seeing a mental image. "Now, you see Him. Do you really—deep down—want to run from Him?"

"No, but in a moment of panic, I might."

"If you know that you do not want God to let go, isn't He wise enough to know that?"

"Yes," Lily laughed ruefully. "That's obvious, isn't it?" Her eyes twinkled with pleasure at the security the thought gave her. Then, switching rapidly, she asked, "Dr. Best, why does Jesus let me hurt so much? The pain would be easier if I had a reason."

"I don't know that answer." Dr. Best turned, looking toward the picture of Christ behind his desk. "I do know that God will not withhold any good thing from you. If you ask honestly, and if it is good for you to know, He will tell you." Then looking directly at Lily, he said matter-of-factly, " Now, I would appreciate your telling me a bit about your background. What was it like when you were growing up?"

"Hell!" Lily blurted out, then bit her lip. "I mean, I was unhappy and confused as a child after I started public school." She surveyed the psychiatrist's face for reaction to her accidental violation of the church language code. There was only honest concern.

"Tell me, did your parents love you?"

"Yes. I was their only child, very special."

"Too special perhaps?" Dr. Best paused, then without waiting for an answer, asked, "Did you like elementary school?"

"I hated it, every minute."

"I'm sure there were good reasons. Did you have trouble with grades? With teachers? Did you have friends?"

Hostility, generated by the recalling of painful memories, was suddenly unleashed upon the doctor. "Look, I've recited those agonies to a dozen other therapists," Lily snapped belligerently, rising up in her chair. "It has never helped. I have always ended up rejected and alone, with someone knowing too much about me. And I don't want to tell you!"

"Lily, have I rejected you yet?" Dr. Best said gently. "Haven't I passed all of your tests?"

"What? How did you know about the tests?" Lily's eyes widened in surprise. "Doctors aren't supposed to know about them."

"I have been at this a long time. And I know a young lady who has learned to be cautious." The psychiatrist shifted into a more authoritarian posture. "Now, tell me about elementary school."

"It was awful. I was always the smartest, always the most polite, always nominated and never chosen, always different."

"Your intelligence and good manners couldn't gain you acceptance from the other children. What about the teachers?"

"In kindergarten my teacher liked to embarrass me. One rainy day, my mother told me to ask the teacher to let me ride home from school with her as far as her house, which was only a block from ours. Mother didn't want me getting wet walking all the way from school and getting a worse cold. My mother didn't drive. When I asked, the teacher looked startled and said, 'what makes you so special? Why should I take just you?' I hid in the playhouse and cried. She made some remark to the class about crybabies.

"In first grade, we had to sit perfectly still in our seats and never get up without permission. I always finished my work early and had nothing to do. I read ahead in my reader until the teacher caught me and made me put it up.

"One day the teacher handed back my *Think-and-Do* reading workbook with the word *DO* written in big red letters at the top of the page. I told her, 'But I did that page.' She said, 'You need to read it.' She meant I needed to read it again and correct the answers, but I didn't understand. I thought she was saying that I lied, that I hadn't read the page. I changed the answer that I thought might be wrong and joined the long line to have the page checked. The teacher said, 'Why did you change that one? I told you to read it again.' From then on, I randomly changed answers and waited for them to be checked. Finally I changed, *did Jane guess?* to *No*. The teacher said, 'Well! You finally did it!'

"That did it for that teacher forever. She had not only implied that I lied—as I understood her—but she was a liar herself. Jane *had* guessed, though not correctly. If I had had any gumption, I would have thrown the book at her and run out the door. I would have been spanked, but that would have been for a real offense. Instead, I was too well mannered. I seethed inside for the rest of the year. The angrier I grew, the more polite I was to her. The more polite I was, the more I hated that teacher. That set a pattern forever. I was always polite; the more I hated an authority, the more polite I became. But at least I obeyed God's commandment to respect and obey authorities."

"Were all your school years so unhappy?" Dr. Best asked frowning.

"Second and third grades were better. The teachers let me learn as much as I wanted and did not make fun of me. But in fourth grade, we moved to Florida. The kids in Florida hated me. I was new, and they let me know daily that I wasn't wanted. Fifth grade was worse. The teacher ridiculed me at every opportunity. She'd hurt my feelings, and when I would cry, she would say to the class, 'Look at the baby.'

"Strange things started happening inside of me then. But I guess they weren't important." Lily fell silent, reluctant to expose any more hurts.

"Go on, Lily," Dr. Best urged gently. "I'm beginning to understand where your problems come from."

"My body began to act so odd. I was growing fast and always hungry. At times, my stomach hurt so bad I would double over. When I played games at school, my arms and legs just wouldn't cooperate, and they hurt, really hurt. Sometimes I would get dizzy and feel like the world was miles away. When I asked adults about this, they would say 'just growing pains.' And—no, never mind."

"What is it?" Dr. Best probed, leaning slightly toward her.

"Well, I never told my other therapists this. But one time a friend asked me to go to a movie matinee for her birthday party. Movies were a rare treat. I can't remember what it was about—or I'm afraid to remember, maybe. Anyhow, a few weeks later, I noticed that the world seemed like a movie, and I was an actress stepping onto the screen."

"Did you tell anyone?"

"No, my parents had their own troubles. Jobs were hard to find, so there wasn't much money. They both seemed upset about things. They hadn't understood about the hunger and pain. So I didn't bother them."

"Did anything else happen that bothered you?"

"Well, I don't know if I should say."

"Trust me."

Lily gazed out the window across the green lawn, and then took a deep breath. Dr. Best had earned her trust; she would risk telling him. "One night, I was getting washed to go to bed. I was alone. A young woman in a green suit suddenly stood in the doorway of the bathroom and said, 'Hello, I'm here to be your sister. I will take you to your real home.' Then she disappeared. I told myself that I certainly had an active imagination, like the adults had always said. But the next day, as I was walking home from school, she and a man, my brother, stepped out from a live oak grove to meet me. That's when all the changes began."

"Changes?"

"Changes in the laws that I lived by. Before, I had lived by the same time/space laws as everyone else. Afterward, everything was different."

"I am not sure I understand. You were not bound to time and space?"

Oh, Dr. Best," Lily's voice wavered. "I shouldn't be talking about these things. I'll pay dearly."

"You'll be all right. Part of your unconscious mind knows you need to talk about this. That part will keep you safe." The psychiatrist spoke with such conviction that his words became reality for Lily, allowing her to feel safe enough to continue the sensitive self-revelation.

She said, "I didn't notice the changes much at first. But in sixth grade, we moved again, this time to a college town. I thought maybe I could make friends. The children were better educated, more cultured, better disciplined, and more open to me. But one day before I left the school building, two boys got in a fight over who would walk me home. When I came out and saw them banged up, I heard the voice of my old Sunday school teacher say, 'Anger is the same as murder.' And I knew I had doomed their souls. From then on, I knew it was dangerous to be my friend."

"So, Lily, social rules seemed to change. Were there other changes?"

Lily marveled at Dr. Best's calm acceptance of her

experience. "Yes, sometimes gravity didn't seem to apply to me, and I would feel as if I was drifting through the air. Several times I awoke and felt myself hovering over my bed; then immediately I landed on it with a thump.

"Time changed. It would have pleats, as I told you before. I would not remember what I had done or said. And sometimes something else took over my body, and I couldn't control it." Lily wrapped her arms around her body protectively. "Once I was in a play pillow fight with some girlfriends. Before I knew what was happening, the 'thing' took over, and I was beating and beating and beating on my best friend. I beat until she was almost unconscious. A few days later, I ripped open her little cousin's arm with my fingernails." Fearfully, Lily shrank into the corner of her chair. "Only, Dr. Best, please understand, I, Lily, didn't do it."

"Lily, relax. Now look at me." He waited until she looked directly at him. "Those things were part of an illness you did not understand. You have repented and God has forgiven you."

Lily's mouth dropped open. "Forgiven, if I couldn't help it?" Other therapists had told her she wasn't responsible, but no one had said she was forgiven and therefore the matter was finished.

"Yes, Christ's blood covers even wrongs which we cannot control. God has forgotten all about those past things. He doesn't hold them against you. Accept that forgiveness. Let those hurts heal."

Quietly, slowly, Lily murmured, "I wish I could."

"You will. I have confidence in you," Dr. Best said matter-of-factly. Then standing up, he concluded, "You have had enough for one session. I will be praying for you this week. Have a good week."

Lily left in awe and admiration, and to her amazement, feeling somewhat relieved of the old guilts.

CHAPTER 23—SICKNESS, NOT USELESSNESS
April 1974

Wednesday evening when Lily arrived home, she called, "Hi, Lena. I'm home."

Willowy and graceful even at the age of forty-two, Lena was stirring a pot of beef and noodles on the stove. "Hello, Lily, how was your day?"

"It was," Lily quipped as she bounced into the kitchen. "Yum, that smells good."

"You're late. Did you see that new doctor again?"

"Uh-huh. As soon as I wash up, I want to talk to you."

Lena ladled the main dish onto their pink Corelle ware plates and finished setting the table. In the two years that Lily had lived with Lena and her young daughter, supper had become a time for sharing and mutual encouragement. Lena found relief from her routine as a factory worker in Lily's perpetually changing experiences. Lily looked to Lena for acceptance, stability, and mature perspective. Tonight, Lena's daughter was away from home, so they could talk freely.

As soon as Lily said the blessing for the food, she turned to her friend. "Lena, how do you feel about my seeing a psychiatrist?"

"You seem to feel better when you come from his office. If he can help, I'm glad."

"But does it bother you to have me living here—or anything. I mean—I am here alone with your only child in the morning after you go to work." Eyes still focused on her mentor, Lily forked up a mouthful of noodles.

"Lily, I trust you. I'm not sure why you think you need a psychiatrist; I can't see that much change in you.

You're upset about losing your job, but that's natural. I was nervous last winter when I was laid off." Lena hesitated, sipping her ice tea. "You're part of the family. We love you. If I can help–"

"Lena, you do help me." Lily interrupted anxiously. "You accept me as I am, and that's what I need. I was afraid my seeing a shrink would scare you, or make you think less of me."

"You had told me that you had problems once before."

"There's a difference between hearing about someone's past and living with a crazy person."

"Oh, Lily, you are not crazy!" Lena laughed. "And pass the green beans."

Passing the pink bowl, Lily asked earnestly, "Be honest with me. How do I act? Do I make sense when I talk? Do I look normal? Can people tell there is anything wrong with me?"

Lena served her own green beans, and then said, "You look tired and discouraged. A little nervous maybe. Otherwise all right."

"Good, then I can still cover up what I think and feel." Lily twirled her noodles around her fork as she talked. "You know, God has been good. He has always allowed a bit of me to stay out of the sickness. It's like a tiny part of me floats over my head watching the rest of me have hallucinations and think sick thoughts. That tiny bit is how I know that some things that are real to me are not real to everyone else. I know better than to talk about the little white worms falling out of the sky or to ask if you can smell my rottenness."

"You really think those things? You don't act like it." Conversation lapsed as Lena considered this new information. Finally she asked, "Lily, you're telling me that you are really sick in your mind, but you can keep from acting like it. Can most people with your problem do that?"

"I'm not sure. I do know that mental illness doesn't have to mean uselessness, worthlessness, if the person will exert his best efforts at control."

"I don't understand. Just a minute, while I get more ice tea. Do you want some?"

"Yes, please." Lily took the freshly filled glass from Lena and set it on a coaster. "If a mentally ill person really works at self-control, she can do most things she could do otherwise. For example, during the first summer that I was in therapy in college, I was really confused. I saw jagged lights around people's heads. I heard noises and voices constantly. But I was determined to stay in school and that meant controlling my actions. To get away from my own problems, I accepted the job of leading our college volunteer program at a correctional school. To my surprise, the girls liked me. My own problems actually helped me understand them."

"So you made your problems work *for* you?" Lena asked, buttering her biscuit.

"Yes. Also the younger college students sensed something about me and trusted me. Before my sickness was generally known on campus, freshmen often opened up their whole lives to me. I tried to talk to them like Prof talked to me. Until the middle of my senior year, I was able to discipline myself, to use the good parts of my mind to help other people. If I could do that, I believe many other mentally ill people can be responsible and useful at least a few hours a day." Lily finished her green beans, and then spoke emphatically. "Mental illness is an illness, not an excuse for irresponsibility."

"Lily, what does this new doctor say?"

"Dr. Best says to regard my experiences as legitimate. He talks about this as a part of my growth toward Christian maturity."

"I think he is right. God has something special for you to do, and you have to go through these things to be ready."

Lily beamed. "Lena, may I tell you a secret? Please don't laugh. When I first knew I was schizie, I wondered if God could use me as an interpreter between the world of mental illness and the normal world. So I've kept a detailed record of my thoughts and experiences and therapy. One day when I was writing and praying, I felt Jesus there with me, and I had the impression that when I have solved my problems, I would be able through writing to encourage other people with serious mental illness and to interpret their world to their therapists and friends. Maybe, Lena, just maybe—"

"Lily, when you are a famous writer and counselor and flying around the country, may I go along as chaperone? Come on. Let's clean up these supper dishes."

Above the clinking of the dishes, the phone rang on the worn wooden desk on the far side of the room. "Lily, would you get the phone? My hands are wet."

Picking up the receiver, Lily heard Warren's deep, steady voice on the line. "Hello, Lily. How are you and Dr. Best getting along?"

"Great, he actually has answers. I miss seeing you though."

"That is why I called. I wonder if you could come to the counseling center tomorrow evening and help me with a child. I have been working with her parents, but I don't know how to get through to the girl."

"What's her problem?"

"She is visually handicapped, ten years old, and very withdrawn. As far as I can tell, she needs someone to build a personal relationship with her. Since you aren't going to be working much longer, I thought you might have time."

"Warren," Lily interrupted, "after you saw me upset two weeks ago, why would you ask me to counsel? How can you trust me?"

"Why shouldn't I trust you?"

"Disturbed people aren't supposed to be counselors."

"You aren't *people*. You are you, and I have always been able to trust you here. How many times have you been in tears in my office, and an hour later I found you at the secretarial desk handling the phone and calming clients as if nothing ever bothered you? In the past you divorced your problems from your work, and I assume you will now. And besides, you will feel better being around the center where you are secure and busy. I will be there if you need me."

"Warren, you're terrific. I'll see you tomorrow at 4:00." Lily gently laid down the receiver and turned to Lena. "Warren wants me to do another counseling case for him. He says he still trusts me. You say you trust me. I don't understand. How can you and Warren and Dr. Best know about my sickness and still trust me?"

"Lily, as far as I can tell, the only person who doesn't trust you is you."

"My bosses haven't trusted me."

"They didn't know the real you. But then maybe that is why you don't trust yourself; you don't really know yourself either."

Late that night Lily lay in bed watching the moonlit shadows play across her ceiling. *Lena trusts me. Warren trusts me. Dr. Best trusts me. I don't trust me. Well, maybe they shouldn't either. But then they don't know that this whole illness is my fault. I wonder if I dare tell Dr. Best.*

CHAPTER 24—GROWING UP
April 1974

"I dare. I dare, I dare," Lily repeated under her breath as she followed Dr. Best from the waiting room into his office.

As she seated herself in the blue wing chair at an angle to Dr. Best's, the psychiatrist looked at her quizzically. "You dare—what?"

Lily blushed. "Oh, I was just working up courage to talk about my past. You wanted to continue where we left off last week, didn't you?"

"That would be helpful to me, but what did *you* want to talk about?"

Lily blushed again. Dr. Best had seen straight through her attempt to place the burden of the hour upon him. She laughed nervously. "The past, I guess. You said that Jesus forgave even guilts we could not control. What would you say if I told you I made the decision that is responsible for my illness?"

"Tell me about it."

Lily briefly described her confusion and pain in tenth grade and what she considered her decision to deal with the pain by separating her emotions from her thinking, just as she had told her first psychologist eight years ago. This time, she concluded, "So I am really responsible for the split in my personality. Therapists can blame my parents, schools, churches, or chemistry, but actually I am responsible."

"I am not certain of that, Lily. You are being hard on yourself."

"Well, I made the decision."

"Was it really a decision or, in fact, a recognition of

what had already happened?" Knowing he was on sensitive territory, Dr. Best kept his voice unemotional, academic, to avoid arousing Lily's unconscious defenses. "You already had a well-developed fantasy system, including an island kingdom, a brother, a sister, and a fantasy-friend Shawn. You simply assigned your emotions to Lily and the rational facets of your personality to Shawn, making Shawn a part of yourself, and pulling your emotions and intellect farther apart. You brought about the logical conclusion to the illness already present." When Lily sighed and gave him a half-smile, seeming somewhat relieved, Dr. Best risked a probing question. "What would have happened if you hadn't made that decision?"

"I don't know. But I think I would have killed myself." Lily paused waiting for the alarm reaction that usually resulted from any mention of suicide. When Dr. Best did not react, she continued. "I know that the weirdness in me would have seeped out repeatedly in the classroom, and my junior and senior years in high school could not have improved."

"You mean there were better years?"

"Now that I think of it, yes. I guess the summer following my sophomore year in high school began the improvement. My mother was spending the summer at a university working on her master's degree. I lived in the dorm with her and took a chemistry class at the experimental high school. I loved the quiet, the library, and the intellectual atmosphere. My achievements and the calm of the summer somehow freed me. I guess I had proved myself in a world that appreciated me."

"Lily, you have always felt you had to prove yourself, and you are still trying. Yet the world is not impressed by your intellect, is it? Intellectual prowess isn't so important in real life. That must be frustrating for you."

Lily stared at the doctor incredulously. *This man is strange. What could be more important than the greatness of one's mind?*

All was quiet until Dr. Best asked, "You said your

last two years of high school improved."

"Thinking of myself as feelingless, like a rock, made it easier for me to get involved in activities. There was less danger of getting hurt. I remember one weekend when our speech club was participating in a state contest on a university campus. We were spending the night in a college dorm. A bunch of us girls were up goofing off long past curfew. One of the girls started demonstrating a dance called the twist. Since our church had convinced me that dancing was a terrible sin, I tried to escape behind a book, but I couldn't concentrate.

"I was shocked when my best friend joined in on such a sensual abomination. Finally I couldn't stand the temptation any longer; I threw down my book and jumped up. "Hey, is this it?" I said, and made a crude attempt at dancing. Everyone laughed. To my dismay, I enjoyed the laughter. In fact I began to enjoy people—I whose theme song was the pop tune about being a rock, an island.

"From then on, I spent less time studying and more time with friends. To my surprise, my grades remained A's. Oddly, the internal pressure eased, and I could learn more readily."

"So you found social acceptance."

"A sort of acceptance. The other kids still considered me 'different', but the difference didn't matter. Actually, during the practices for our senior class play, I became sort of a 'Dear Abby'. I did pretty well for the other kids, but, oh, the pain for me."

"Pain?" questioned Dr. Best. "Tell me what happened."

"My best friend my senior year was a foreign refugee. She had been through horrible things." Lily sighed, vividly remembering her friend's distress. "She told me about them, about her present nightmares, her fears, and how she fought impulses to hurt herself. She was too scared to go to the mental health clinic and wanted me to help her. I often threw around psychological jargon as if I were an expert, but a problem like my friend's scared me. But since she wouldn't talk to anyone else, I thought I had to try. I dug into my mother's college psychology textbooks and was horrified that the problem was considered so serious. However my friend was depending on me so I wouldn't give up. She and I discussed over and over what had happened to her, her present conflicts and pressures, and various means of relieving frustration. I talked to her about Jesus. After each session, my friend felt better, but the improvement never lasted." Tears stood in Lily's eyes.

"Finally one evening we sat in my car talking, parked by the lake where we wouldn't be interrupted. I was almost as desperate as she was. I blurted out, 'Look, Jesus, my friend can't get any relief, and she can't seem to understand about You. But I know You, and as Your friend I'm asking You, please take these problems away from her. Heal her. Thank You.' Dr. Best, you know what? He did. Within a few months, my friend was happier." Lily was laughing.

Then, as other memories streamed into Lily's consciousness, she turned pale. "My friend was okay, but I wasn't. After what I had found in the books, I was thoroughly scared."

"What were you afraid of? What had you read?"

"Until I had studied those books, I had shrugged off my split as a joke, a trick I was playing on myself, one that I could stop at any time. I assumed that everyone had the same kind of sensory experiences that I did." Lily shuttered.

"What you read changed your mind?"

"Yes. Do you have any idea how it feels to read through a book, to come upon the title *schizophrenia*, and find yourself described under it? For a high school senior, it is quite a shock."

"That would be a shock at any age. What exactly did you read?"

"I don't remember. That was many books ago. I know what bothered me most was the description of sensory experience—detached from surroundings, the world looking flat and unreal, faces and objects pulsating and changing shapes, hands feeling distant and small, a conviction of being overpowered by an unknown force. Those things had been a regular part of my life ever since fifth grade. Also, I had attacks in which I would throw everything in sight and scream and cry, but since I could postpone those attacks until I was alone, I had rationalized that I was in control. My reading proved I was not."

"What did you do then?"

"I used to walk past the mental health clinic, yearning to go in, but not daring. I knew the clinic would tell my parents and spoil my image of being perfect. My greatest hope was that once I was in college, a change in environment would be the solution."

"What happened when you went to college?"

"I didn't get to find out for a while. The day—Dr. Best, why in the world am I telling you all of this? It is irrelevant to my present problem, and I would be better off not talking about it."

Lily felt herself shaking inside. If she were to explain about her father's illness, she would have to expose a tender part of herself that she could not afford to have misunderstood. She had never told other therapists, and she was not sure she trusted even Dr. Best quite that far.

Dr. Best gently prompted her. "Past experience often shapes present perspective. I wish you would trust me to accept what you were about to say."

Lily saw a soft glow on Dr. Best's face. *The light of love,* she thought. *I'll take the risk.*

"The day I was supposed to leave for college, my father was operated on for cancer. After the surgery, the doctor gave him only until Christmas to live. The cancer had spread too far to be controlled or removed."

"That must have been difficult to hear. How did it affect you?" Lily heard a sudden concern in his voice that was more than professional and wondered why.

"I listened coolly and walked out of the hospital. When I was out of sight, lost in the autumn drizzle, I cried until there were no more tears to cry. Then I told God exactly what I thought of Him for doing that to my father and to me—and what I said wasn't nice. But Jesus understood, as He always does, and wrapped me up in His love. I walked calmly back into the hospital and told my mother to go home, that I would stay with my father. In the tiny hospital, the family often did part of their own nursing. I stayed up with my father all night."

"Were you always so in control?" Dr. Best asked in puzzlement.

"That night I was. I had business to finish with God, and I intended to take care of it promptly and efficiently. While I was waiting for my father to go to sleep, I overheard the nurses questioning whether he would live through the night. That solidified my plans. As soon as he was asleep, I slipped into the bathroom and closed the door so that I would not be heard.

" 'Now listen, God,' I said. 'It isn't fair to keep my father alive in such pain—fair to him or to me. Either heal him and let him have a healthy life for ten years, or let him die tonight. That is the arrangement I want between us, and I won't give up until I get it. You said that the effectual, fervent prayer of a righteous man will be answered. I am righteous because of the Cross, and this prayer is fervent enough that I won't give up until You say *yes.*' Then I reminded God of at least a dozen Scripture passages on His faithfulness and answered prayer."

"And what happened?" Dr. Best asked, not disguising the deep concern in his voice.

"My father lived through the night. He had many other surgeries and was sick for several years. But today he is alive, ten years later, and well and happier than I have ever known him to be."

"So God chose to answer you."

"Look, Dr. Best, when I pray like that night, He has to say *yes*—because I can't pray that way unless He gives me the power for it in the first place." Lily's voice rose in defensive irritation. She slid forward in the wing chair until she was almost standing. "According to my friend, Rev. Dopson, that is the prayer of faith talked about in James 5. I know many people don't believe miracles happen today, but I wish they would keep their doubts to themselves."

"Lily, relax. I understand. You know a special kind of prayer that few people experience. I respect that."

Surprised at his acceptance of her pronouncements, Lily relaxed and sat back in her chair. "Did you go on to college?"

"No, I stayed home and took care of my father. I was much better prepared to deal with his day-to-day medical problems than my mother was, and she needed to continue teaching so that we had some income."

Dr. Best gave her a warm, approving smile. "When did you start college?"

"Second semester. God had kept His word." Lily smiled at the memory. "In January of 1965, a month after my father should have been dead, he drove me to college. It was a small, evangelical liberal arts school about four hundred miles from home."

"How did you get along there?"

"For the first time in my life, I felt that I truly belonged. I fit in with the students and soon made lots of friends. I held several leadership positions. What I said carried importance with the other students. Within a short time, the professors respected me too. I loved that school until the end of my sophomore year, but by that time the illness had overpowered me so that I could not love anything."

"You started in psychotherapy with the college psychologist that spring?"

"Yes, but could we talk about that another time? I'm going to pay a high price for exposing this much."

Dr. Best accepted Lily's diversion with a smile that said, *I see your tactic but I understand why you need it.*

"Perhaps then this is an appropriate time to ask you what you thought about the book on the role of nutrition in symptoms like some of yours."

"I thought it made sense," Lily said, sliding comfortably into an attitude of academic discussion. "Especially the section about abnormal reactions to foods causing sensory disturbances. In the winter, my physical symptoms are always worse. And in the winter, I always eat a lot of oranges and other foods the book mentions as causing problems for some people. I mean, oranges are supposed to be healthy, right? The year I was so disturbed at college, I often ate two oranges a day. But when I was very young, I would break out in hives if I ate orange juice or mint flavoring. I thought I had outgrown those allergies. The book suggests that sensitivity shows up in different forms over time. But how would that work?"

"These theories are fairly new. They are based on observations that clinicians have made more than on medical research. As a treatment, nutritional therapy is still trial and error."

"I'm involved in the trial; I hope there is no error," Lily laughed.

"Explain." Dr. Best waved his hand in a gesture that indicated he was becoming accustomed to Lily's obscure speech.

"I've started not eating anything in the salicylate food group and I'm adding in one vitamin. It makes sense that changing what goes into the body would change how the body functions. I would rather use nutrition than medication."

"Lily," Dr. Best interrupted in a worried tone. "I hope that doesn't mean you have abruptly stopped taking the anti-psychotic medication you have been using all this time."

"No, I know more biochemistry than to do that. Nutritional therapy is an addition, not a substitution."

"Yes, of course." Dr. Best took a deep breath of relief. "I should have known that about you." He looked at his watch. "It is getting late." He stood up, signaling the end of the session. As he escorted her toward the waiting room, he commented, "I'll look forward to what you have to tell me next week. I think we have a relationship of trust."

That night in her room, after she had pulled on her red fleece pajamas and settled herself cross-legged on her bed, Lily began to write in her journal. "I have trusted Dr. Best with that which I have entrusted to no other therapist, and he has not misunderstood. Could it be that there is one man who can be totally trusted with one's being? He has seen through every diversion, by-passed every defense. I have always felt that if I could entrust myself wholly and unreservedly to one person whom I respected and that one person loved me for myself and did not reject or run from me, then I could trust myself. Then I could trust and interact with people, instead of having to manipulate them for my own protection. I could really be free.

"But that kind of trust necessitates that the other person see me as a person, not a patient. This man is a doctor; he is only doing his job for his patient. I am supposed to see him as a professional, not a person, and to relate to him within the rules.

"Dear God, that is hard. Every time I look at Dr. Best, I forget he is a professional. I forget he is only performing a role and I, a role. I see a real man with a heart of love and warmth and acceptance—all that I want in a special friend. Jesus, I want to know Louis, not the doctor. But I know my feelings are against the rules.

"Even worse, God, is the distinct feeling that he sees me as a person, not just a patient. From the moment I met him, I felt a special bond, like You had ordained the meeting."

Lily listened silently for Jesus' voice, and then wrote, "You ask, what would Dr. Best say if he read this. He would say, 'How can I help you if you don't tell me? I am worthy; I have passed your tests. Trust me. Trust me.'"

CHAPTER 25—TRUST RESTORED
April 1974

"Trust me. Trust me," reverberated through Lily's head as she seated herself in her usual blue wing chair in Dr. Best's plush office.

All right, she screamed mentally. *I'll trust this man. I'll say what I really think. But, God, if Dr. Best reacts like most of those other Christians, You'd better be prepared to meet me at the state mental hospital.*

After the preliminary formalities, Lily braced herself. She must express her feelings now; she would never have the courage again.

"Dr. Best, you have answered more questions for me than anyone else. You make sense. I don't often say that about doctors. But there is something you don't know, and I'm afraid to tell you."

"I can take it." Dr. Best smiled his prepared-for-anything smile. "What is bothering you?"

Lily gripped the chair arms and braced herself to be mentally destroyed. "I *like* you."

"Is that bad?" Dr. Best sounded genuinely puzzled.

"Yes, I'm supposed to regard you simply as a professional. But I see you as a person. That's wrong."

"I told you it was all right to feel anything you want in this office. Tell me what you like about me." Dr. Best held the smile steady, but it was not quite that bland professional smile.

Lily blushed. "You understand me. You accept me. You have a kind, soft voice. You don't hide your feelings very well; probably you'd be criticized for personal involvement by my counseling professors. You love Jesus. You don't think I'm crazy for saying I know Him. You're just—just real."

Lily stared at the floor. What would be the price of her honesty?

"Well, that is quite a compliment." The corner of the psychiatrist's mouth twitched humorously.

"You're not angry?"

"Why should I be?" The last remnants of his professional mask dropped away. He chuckled deeply. "I admit that earlier in my practice that could have been hard to handle. But I've grown to the point that I know whatever I am is from God. And He is the One who sends people to me. Thank Him for the warmth you feel."

"Well, if you can accept that, I guess I can tell *you* anything!" Relief ran through Lily's whole body. She had given the ultimate confidence, the vulnerability for him to destroy her. He had neither lashed out at her nor retreated from her. He could be trusted and believed. What he told her about herself and the world would be solid and true.

"Dr. Best, I've told you about my past. By now, you must know that two weeks ago when I said that I am different, I was right." Shadows and tiny points of light from the window flickered across Lily's face and caught in her eyes: she rubbed her eyes to clear away the irritation.

"You have told me about experiences that are frequent among people with your background and sensitivity," Dr. Best said.

"But I am different. It sticks out all over. In my jobs, my ideas are inevitably different from those of other staff members. In teaching, I relate differently to the children, though they like me. Even when I walk through a department store, people look at me as if I were from outer space."

"Lily, I suspect that it's not what you are but what you do. You expect to be different. You expect people to notice you. So you unconsciously do things to draw attention to yourself. Maybe your dress, your speech, your facial expressions, your walk."

Catching the idea, Lily laughed. "I see what you

mean. Maybe it's my 'I'm free' attitude. There is a television actress who runs, skips, and flies kites. When I'm out shopping and I'm happy, I often pretend I am she. I guess she does make herself pretty conspicuous. But I enjoy skipping and smiling at everyone. I don't feel so ultra-bookish then."

"Lily, you don't have to act like you did as a preschooler to be happy and you don't have to imitate anyone else. Are you afraid to be a normal person?"

Lily grinned sheepishly. "I guess so. I'm afraid if I am ordinary, I'll cease to exist—you know, all those magazine articles about being lost in the crowd."

"Lily, you are doing it again," Dr. Best chuckled, crossing his legs comfortably. "You take exaggerated generalizations and apply them to yourself. Don't worry; try as hard as you may, you can never be lost in a crowd. Your basic personality will keep you safe, and sooner or later your talents will be noticed."

Dr. Best's explanation was lost in the sudden rumbling of Lily's internal volcano. The inner turmoil must have shown through because Dr. Best asked, "Lily, what is the matter?"

Now that she had given herself to Dr. Best, her disturbance forced itself into the relationship. She needed a safety valve for the repressed violence inside her and in this office she knew she would not be misunderstood.

Dramatically, Lily's face contorted; her eyes narrowed into slits. She intoned, "I don't want to be like people. I hate people. I hate every one of them and everything about them." Tears of anguish followed the stinging words.

Leaning forward intently, Dr. Best probed, "Do you hate me?"

"You're a man. That doesn't count?"

"Men aren't people? It is women you don't want to be like? What about the woman psychiatrist you have talked about?" countered Dr. Best.

"She is different. I love her. So is my Aunt Violet.

They don't go around chasing men, with a couple of babies under each arm, and squabbling over who makes the best hors d'oeuvres, scheming to stab each other in the back—and all the while letting the men lord it over them. No, I'm not like them. I won't be! I--."

"God doesn't want you to be!" Dr. Best spoke sharply, penetrating the torrent of verbiage. Lily stopped and stared at him. "God does not want you or any other woman to be what you just described."

"But that is what they are. I watched and I listened."

"Who? Where? Give me names and places."

"Well—." Blank. For five minutes Lily looked off into space, her mind racing through the void. No names, no places, yet a distinct image. Perhaps a composite. Then darkness.

"Lily, is that your mother?" Dr. Best's voice trickled through her concentration. She tried desperately to answer.

"No," she whispered. "Nothing like her. Women at church, Sunday school teachers said, 'Don't be like other women.' Parties, gossip circles. Teachers at school said, 'When you get married, don't--.' I don't know. I don't--." She pounded her knee with her fist. "I can't see you. You're too far away."

"It's all right. You're afraid of the unknown, so you're shutting out the world. Your woman is a stereotype, not real, probably pieces of conversation you have heard and believed when you were young. You picked all the stereotypical faults and made them into a person."

Not sure if he was being heard, Dr. Best spoke distinctly. "You—are—not—to—be—that—kind—of—human. Can you hear me?" He repeated the statement.

Finally Lily answered, "Yes, you're getting closer."

"You told me that you promised yourself never to be a typical teenager like you overheard the older ladies gossiping about. Is that the root of your image of a woman? Those gossips were big; you were little. You took them literally. Lily, they were just talking to have something to say. Your image is not real."

As Dr. Best's words soaked in, Lily could see his face again. He handed her a brown paperback book. "Study this and read Proverbs 31 from a modern translation. The ideal woman in Proverbs is an organizer, a businesswoman, an artist, a provider, and thoroughly competent. And what you are really reacting against is a picture of women as dependent and incompetent. Lily, God made you competent in many areas. He gave you a desire for independence. Accept that and be thankful."

The conversation drifted for a while and then Lily glanced at the list of questions in the notebook on her lap. "There is one other important question," she said. "Why does God treat me differently from other people? I did what I was taught in Sunday school. But I ended up hating God for making me sinful and evil and then ordering me to be good. I believed my college's description of God. I tried the 'surrender yourself' and the 'be crucified with Christ,' all the formulas, to get the joy and peace the other students had, but the formulas didn't work for me."

Dr. Best paused, and then asked pointedly. "You have had many false ideas and fantasies. How do you know that your relationship with Jesus isn't another fantasy?"

Lily's eyes widened in surprise. To her, the question was ludicrous. How could she explain the impossible? Hesitantly she said, "I told you about the answers I've had to prayers. That was not fantasy. I can document it." Seeing that Dr. Best was accepting her reasoning, she continued. "But there is another way. When I was first diagnosed as schizophrenic, I kept a detailed journal to check my reality against the other students' reality. I found that the more I lived in social and physical reality, the more real Jesus was. The more I lived in fantasy or was mentally confused, the less I could communicate with Him.

"Dr. Best, the only reason I have stayed alive and tried to get well is because Jesus wants me to. But so many preachers say we only know Jesus through the Bible. I can't understand the Bible because of my mixed-up past.

But I do know Jesus."

"That kind of difference I wish more people had," Dr. Best said, smiling broadly.

"I don't understand. You wish more people were abnormal?"

"No. Let's sort out what you said. First, being different isn't always being bad. Second, you say you are different because you know Jesus personally, as a personality with likes, dislikes, angers, loves. That's bad? Then Abraham, Moses, the Apostles and the church fathers were bad. Third, when preachers insist on our knowing God only through the Bible, they are talking about an objective revelation of truth. Without the written revelation, you would not have known how to get acquainted with Jesus, right?" Lily nodded. "Preachers are also trying to avoid the cults and other religions that have ideas contrary to the Bible. Has your Jesus ever shown you anything contrary to Scripture?"

"No! No! Jesus shows me personal things, like choosing a college or a job—or a dress." Lily grinned sheepishly, thinking of her prayers during recent shopping trip and the pleasing results. "The Bible doesn't tell me what practical decisions to make, and usually I'm too confused to decide for myself."

"Then thank Him for communicating with you. That difference is to be respected." Dr. Best looked out the window into the blue heavens for a few moments, then turned back toward Lily and said, "You've mentioned being confused by theological controversies before. Scripture leaves room for some variation in interpretation and for different ways of stating the same truth. A few of those interpretations have played into your weaknesses. I'm sorry about that."

Lily couldn't believe her ears. This doctor was sorry? She leaned forward on the arm of the chair, listening closely as Dr. Best explained.

"In spite of the variations, the Bible has one central, clear message. God so loved this world that, as Jesus, He came to Earth. He lived like we do. He allowed Himself to be crucified to pay for our sins and to defeat evil. He was resurrected. He is in Heaven loving us and reaching out to us today."

"No magic words to be said?" To Lily, the catch phrases in churches had sounded like words with magical, mystical meanings.

"No special words, no! Your confusion over language must have made what you heard in various churches sound like different gospels. I suspect that some non-Christians feel the same way. Lily, your relationship with God is valid, even if you don't use the theological words. Accept it and be thankful. Hang in there. You are a remarkable young lady."

Lily left the office in awe. She had trusted and survived. She had exposed all her differences, her weaknesses, and her weirdness; yet Dr. Best had not glossed over, rejected, deceived, or emotionally fled from her. He believed in her.

If Dr. Best believed in her, then perhaps she should believe in herself. Since he loved her with agape love and it had no ill effect on him, perhaps she dared to love herself. She had said that to trust entirely was to be healed. Well?

CHAPTER 26—THANK GOD, I'M SCHIZIE
April 1974

Secluded in her cold, dingy-yellow office at the state institution for the retarded early Thursday afternoon, Lily shuffled through the piles of papers on her desk. Gingerly she fingered a large manila envelope newly arrived in the mail. "I wonder what is in this envelope from the psychology department office? Some kind of time bomb?"

Tearing open the flap, Lily pulled out a duplicated set of her last resident reports, and a hand-written memo from the department head. She starred at the reports. *It seems like months ago that I wrote these, instead of two weeks. I wonder why the note from the department head. What's gone wrong now?*

Lily read silently, "Dear Lily, these reports are informative, well-written, and display an understanding of the needs of the severely retarded. I am sorry that you will no longer be with our department. However, the unit feels you do not fit its needs. Personally, I believe that leaving this position will be best for you in the long run. I will be glad to recommend you for a graduate program or another position more suited to your personal and intellectual talents. Sincerely, JCC"

"Well, thank you, JCC," Lily jeered aloud, glaring at the memo in cold, stony hatred. The note, intended to compliment and encourage, had played into Lily's greatest weakness, triggering a psychotic reaction. "Talents, oh, I'm so talented. Smart, oh so smart. So smart, and so talented, I don't fit anywhere. I don't fit here. I didn't fit in teaching. I didn't fit in the lab. I didn't fit in my parents' church. After so long, I didn't even fit on the psych ward. I couldn't even go crazy like other people.

"It seems I don't belong in this world. For eight years it has consigned me to a living hell. 'Keep her alone,' it said. 'Let her burn up in her own pain. Maybe fire will melt the stone,' it said. But there is a way out of this living hell, and maybe I ought to take it. The way out of hell is into heaven."

Rationality temporarily suspended, Lily's hand produced a book of matches from her desk drawer. Without feeling or fear, she passed the tip of a burning match back and forth over the length of her bare forearm.

"Hell to heaven.
Count to seven.
Jesus knows.
Here it goes."

Using match after match, she raked the visible symbol of hell and release against the white flesh of her arms. Then pushing back from the desk, she passed the fire across the bare skin of her lower legs until she reached the hem of her madras cotton skirt.

Now the clothes, the hair, the heavens.

Rationality seized her; she hurled the matches across the room. "No, God, no. Stop me!"

Frantically she picked up the phone and dialed Dr. Best's number. "Please, Dr. Best, help me. I want to burn the world and myself. This is Lily and I can't stand the pain. You think I can handle myself... Call you tomorrow? All right. Pray for me. Good-bye."

Incapable of remaining rational under the internal pressure, yet unwilling to betray Dr. Best's confidence in her, Lily used her last escape. She slid her body under the kneehole of her desk and mentally evaporated. About 3:00 p.m., Lily re-entered the world as Shawn, the queen who guards the secrets of the worlds. Shawn glanced disgustedly at the book of matches on the floor but picked them up and slipped them into her purse for future reference. She looked at her reddened arms. *Nothing serious, I can treat them later. The sooner I'm out of the depressing building, the better for my head.* She signed out early and walked to her Chevy.

Once on the open road, she headed for a wooded lane, hoping to find calmness and rest in the drive. Lecturing herself aloud, she said, "Really, I should never allow myself to be solely Lily. That fragile flower has no perspective. I need to consistently remind myself that I am Shawn—pronounced with a soft Southern "ah" like the Shawnandoah River for which I am named—and I carry the strength and dignity of that river.

"Imagine—the two times I dared mention my name as Shawn, the therapists chided me for having a male name, like Sean in the movies. Dolts! I tried to explain, and then realized that bearing the name of a river would not fit their psychological schemes. Therapists can be so dense. I wonder if all mankind appears equally numbskull to God."

Lily paused, hearing Shawn's words. She laughed at their arrogance and artificiality. "I'm being ridiculous, what my third grade teacher would call 'Riding my high horse.' I think God would like for me to get off that horse. Sorry, Jesus."

Driving slowly, Lily glanced appreciatively at the new spring greenery, at the maple and hickory trees shadowing the lane, and scented the perfume of the lilacs blooming along the road.

"Jesus, as long as I am apologizing to You, I might as well bring up an issue that has been bothering me. In reading my old journals, I marvel at what I could do in my lucid moments during college—and like most schizoids, I had more rational hours than irrational ones. I could do excellent academic work, encourage my friends, cheer up the children at the hospital, and reach the girls at the reform school. If I could achieve, and could love, and could counsel in spite of my sickness, what could I have done if I had been well?

"Remember, I intended to be a doctor because I enjoyed applying science and I wanted to help people? Earning an M.D. is a lost cause now. I failed you. I failed other people. I'm sorry. But I would have succeeded as a doctor if I hadn't been sick. With my intellectual ability, I could have mastered any specialty I chose." The pitch of her voice began to rise. She slowed the car to a crawl. "I could have been an outstanding medical missionary or a prominent pediatrician in New York. I would have had to answer to no one, to bow and scrape to no one. They would have said, " 'Yes, Dr. Farmer,' and 'No, Dr. Farmer', 'As you will, Dr. Farmer.' I have the brains and the determination, and you know it. So, God, why—why did you make me sick?"

Haughty anger again stilted her voice. "Why did you create me so talented and then prevent me from using those gifts? What kind of a God are you?"

Like distant thunder, the familiar Scriptural words describing Jesus rolled across Lily's mind. *He was a man of sorrows and acquainted with grief.... He was despised and rejected. He was wounded for our transgressions; He was bruised for our iniquities: the chastisement of our peace was upon Him: and with His stripes we are healed...Foxes have holes, the birds of the air have nests, but the Son of Man has nowhere to lay His head.* The gentle inner voice added, *Lily, you said you wanted to be like me.*

Lily steered her car to the edge of the lane and parked. Before her hung a mental picture of herself in a handsome red suit, her curls in perfect order, presiding behind an enormous desk. Several renowned physicians took notes as she delivered a lecture on the effects of parental attitude upon chronically ill children. In the fashionable outer office, the secretary spoke insistently into the telephone, "I'm sorry. I understand your daughter is critical and that she is Dr. Farmer's patient. I realize your wife is beside herself. But Dr. Farmer is lecturing, and she is much too important to stop her work for a child. Call back later. Good-bye." When the lecture concluded, the eminent doctors rose. One said, "Brilliant research, Farmer. Gentlemen, will you join me for lunch? Farmer, I assume you have work to do as usual. Good day." Dr. Lillian Farmer leaned against her desk—respected, renowned, and alone—too arrogant to be included, too important to love a dying child.

"Oh, Jesus, no!" Lily burst into tears, cradling her head against the steering wheel. "So remote from people. So good I'm worthless; a brilliant, intellectual snob." She caught her breath, sighed, and relaxed.

"God, if You had given me my way, that would have happened, wouldn't it—if not in New York, then wherever I went. I would a thousand times rather be schizie and be able to love a few Joans and Rebeccas, to befriend a few neglected children. I'd rather be a failure so that in my better moments I could be like Jesus. God, thank you I'm schizie."

The evening sun filtered through the trees, tracing patterns of gold and orange across Lily's arms. Birds in the woods sang their evening chorus of praise. She laughed. "It's a good world, God. You're a good God. At least I'm not a gilded Lily. Let's go home."

CHAPTER 27—THE MEANING OF SUFFERING
April 1974

Not a gilded Lily, but a shrinking violet, Lily reflected, concerning her fear as she followed Dr. Best into his office on the following Wednesday. She scowled as she seated herself in the blue wing chair facing the window. *Trust demands I tell him about my experience in the lane last Thursday; common sense asks, what if he rejects it as crazy? He has passed all of the tests so far, but what about the absurd?* Fingering the velvety chair arm, Lily stared meditatively at the psychiatrist in his easy chair beside the window.

"Lily, you look a little worried," Dr. Best broke into her thoughts.

Lily spoke carefully. "I am. Something happened that I should tell you, something beautiful. But sometimes the telling of beauty is its undoing."

"I enjoy hearing about beautiful things."

Unsure about his meaning, Lily checked the psychiatrist's face for the dreaded counselor's mask: her eyes widened in surprise. *That light on his face! It is that special Light! The Light I saw on Pastor David's in the church sanctuary. And on Rev. Dopson's face. Like a nimbus. A sign that it's safe to tell him.* She took a deep breath and began.

"I'll try to explain what happened," she said, trying to suppress the emotion from her voice. " Last Thursday after I called you, I couldn't fight the fire any longer. So I blacked out. When I came to, I was Shawn, totally Shawn—angry, aloof, cold, and rational. I left work early and drove out into the country. I was yelling at God about my illness and lack of achievement when I saw—well, something happened so that I knew God was there. When it was over, I knew there was a reason He had let me be sick."

"You mean as in Romans 8:28, 'we know that all things work together for good to them that love God.' Certainly there was a reason." He paused. When Lily did not respond, he prompted, "You saw some sort of mental image that explained that reason?"

"You're not surprised? Not going to call it a hallucination?"

"No, certainly not. Tell me about it." The tenderness in Dr. Best's eyes melted the restraining stony fear in Lily's heart.

"I saw what I would have been like if I hadn't been sick, if I had been able to finish medical school and had succeeded professionally. Dr. Best, it was frightening. I was so totally consumed with my own ideas, my respectability, and my brilliance that I couldn't relate to the very people I had trained to serve. After that, I'm actually thankful I'm schizie."

"Lily, are you saying that your illness kept you from the sins of pride, self-righteousness, and arrogance?" Dr. Best picked up a Bible from the lamp table and let it fall open to hand-written notes, deliberately giving Lily time to reflect. When she nodded assent, he continued, "Then you understand what Peter meant in First Peter 4:1 and 2 when he wrote that whoever has suffered physically having the mind of Christ is done with sin—has stopped pleasing himself and the world, and tries to please God."

"Yes," Lily answered slowly. "I think maybe that is it. Because I was blocked from normal life and had to rely on God for ordinary things, I couldn't afford to be arrogant. So it became natural to love the lonely child, the hurting young person, the social reject." She shifted uneasily in her chair: emotion threatened to break through her careful surface. "But there's more to it. I can identify with people with deep problems. You know I have done a lot of informal counseling and some work in Warren's counseling center. When most counselors say, 'I understand,' any disturbed person knows that's a farce. But when I say 'I understand', it is true, or else I won't say it. Disturbed people know the difference."

"Lily, that reminds me of Paul's statement that we suffer so that we may later be able to comfort others with the same comfort with which we were comforted." [II Corinthians 1:3&4]

Lily chewed her lip. *That is what Rev. Dopson said. A second opinion is confirmation.* Aloud she said, "Dr. Best, you use the Bible so differently from other people—well, at least most other authorities. At college and at the churches I attended when I was growing up, they used the Bible to condemn me. I wasn't right in some way—not perfect enough, not happy enough, too inquisitive, too angry, always something. You make the Bible sound like it relates to my experience, like the writers understand me."

"Of course it relates to your experience. The Bible was written by sensitive, seeking individuals like you." Dr. Best kept his voice academic, controlling the anticipation he felt. This rigid, world-wary girl for whom he had prayed so diligently was at the verge of discovery, but any emotion from him could arouse her defenses.

"Then maybe this won't sound conceited to you. I have wanted to tell someone. When I was a child, I thought Abraham was the greatest man in the Old Testament because God called him *friend.* When I was little, I told God the greatest thing He could do for me was to let me be His friend. Dr. Best, if God hadn't let me be sick, when I was grown I would have stuck my self-sufficient nose in the air, turned on my heel, and walked away from Him."

"But now you can say with Paul that you have lost everything in this world that you may know Christ." [Philippians 3:8]

A smile spread across Lily's face. "Yes, I guess I can." She paused to absorb the pleasing realizations about herself. "Dr. Best, I feel almost good about myself when I'm with you. I feel less guilty, stronger, and more able to control my own life. It's like a saying of one of my psychology professors —'Unconditional acceptance with positive regard leads to self-determination.' You give me permission to be." Lily's fingers fidgeted along the arm of the chair.

"God gives you permission to be. Why shouldn't I?"

"My secular therapists did. But too many Christians want me to conform to some mold, some pattern I don't even understand."

"There are no molds, no patterns in this office. You can feel anything here," he said, watching Lily's green eyes dance with excitement.

"If it's okay to feel anything here, does that mean that human emotions are basically good?" She had waited so long to test this idea on someone who could be trusted to understand and tell her the truth. In a moment, she would know for certain.

"Lily, you are leading up to something," Dr. Best grinned. "What is it?"

"I've been thinking about this for a long time. As a child, I was constantly told, directly or indirectly, that emotions are bad, sinful. I was a highly emotional, sensitive child. I thought that if my emotions were wrong and shouldn't exist, then I shouldn't exist either. Without understanding what I was doing, I began destroying that person who should not have existed—and came close to succeeding in doing it. But then in college, when Pastor David, Rebecca, and Dr. Willoughby, and the medical students insisted I had a right to my feelings, all of my feelings, I began to think I had a right to be. So I started to live a little more in reality. At the Catholic college, the nuns valued me for me, and I lived in reality most of the time. And, Dr. Best, you know me. You know I can never be like other people; my difference won't go away. But you accept me. I think I am beginning to accept myself. That means accepting my emotions.

"I got sick partly because I thought emotions were

bad; I get better when I regard emotions as good. From there on, it is just basic math." Lily watched the psychiatrist for any signs of the closed-in clinical mask.

"Math? Would you please explain?" Dr. Best asked, making no attempt to hide his perplexity.

Lily laughed. "If A=B and C=B, then A=C. So, if 'emotions as good (A)' promotes 'health (B)', and if 'truth (C)' promotes 'health (B)', then 'emotions as good' must be 'true' (A=C). Human emotions are basically good. Am I right, Dr. Best?" Knowing full well that rules for *equals* in mathematics might not apply to other relationships in logic, Lily tilted her head and gave the psychiatrist a sideways smile. She believed her point was valid and intended to stick with it.

Dr. Best paused and gazed searchingly at the open Bible on his lap. From Lily's expression, he knew something was amiss in her paradigm, but, being more concerned with helping Lily discover truths she needed than with formal logic, Dr. Best decided to pursue similar reasoning. In an authoritative, academic tone, he asked, "Who created emotions, Lily?"

"God."

"Does God create evil?"

"No. Evil is not a created or self-existent thing. It is a distortion of good. I already know that much."

Dr. Best finished his paradigm. "Then, if God created emotions, and God cannot create evil, then emotions cannot be basically evil. If emotions cannot be evil, then they must be basically good."

Lily stared out the window for a moment, smiled, and let out a long sigh of happiness. Then, with a hint of mischievousness in her voice, she said, "Now comes the tricky part. If emotions are good, then hate can be good. I suspected that a long time ago. I just wasn't sure until now." Dr. Best raised his eyebrows quizzically. Lily laughed and continued, "You see, during my last year at the Christian college, hate, violence, and stubbornness were my major driving forces. Without them, I would have lain down and died. They were mechanisms, however faulty, for preserving a child of God."

Dr. Best stared into the distance, thinking, and then continued methodically. "Well, let's follow your reasoning. The Bible says that God hates evil. So God has hate. And God is all good. Therefore, hate must be good when properly used. Is that what you mean?"

"Yes," Lily's voice was abruptly agitated. Her fist pounded the chair arm. "I hated people I felt were trying to destroy me. That connects hate with self-respect and--."

"Lily, stop!" the psychiatrist commanded, rising up in his chair. "You are falling into the Enemy's trap. STOP!" He saw the danger in her reasoning but for a few moments was uncertain how to guide her.

For those moments, the room was silent. Lily sensed Dr. Best praying fervently and felt the calming presence of Jesus' Spirit surrounding her. Like a chastened little child, she stared at the scuffed toes of her loafers and sat very still. As Lily's mind settled down, Dr. Best asked quietly, "Did you really hate those people?"

"It felt like hate," she murmured.

"Yes, it would feel that way." Dr. Best turned toward the picture of Christ hanging behind his desk. Softly as though talking to himself, he reflected, "Unhealed hurt generates anger. Anger mixed with guilt produces hate. Hate mixed with inferiority feelings produces bitterness." Then looking directly at Lily, he said, "You felt like you hated certain people. But hate means you would enjoy having something terrible happen to them. Would you?"

Mentally, Lily ran through the list of people whom she thought she hated. "I could have gladly thrown something at any of them, or told them exactly what I thought of them. But I wouldn't have wanted any of them to be permanently injured in a car accident, or to get some horrible disease. Or anything like that." Lily stared out the window, trying to reorient her thinking. Her fingers drummed on the arm of the chair. Then she asked. "So are you saying that I did not hate them?"

"You've told me about some of those people. Wasn't it more a matter of being confused by them? And often of trying ineffectively to protect yourself?"

"I guess what I really wanted was for them to go away and leave me alone. Like Prof Filbert. When he hurt me so badly by misunderstanding and accusing me and subtly threatening me, I would have nothing to do with him. I wouldn't even speak to him when I passed him on the sidewalk. It felt like I hated him. But I wouldn't have wanted anything bad to happen to him. In fact, I defended him to other students. Now, I would enjoy seeing him since I'm not in college and he can't do anything to me. Dr. Best, do you mean that everything that feels like hate isn't?"

"Not in your case."

Lily wriggled in child-like excitement. This was too wonderful to believe. "So all these years I thought I was guilty of the sin of hating people, and there was nothing I could do about it, but actually I wasn't hating at all. I was just trying to avoid being hurt again." She thought a minute. Engaging her quick powers of reasoning again, she extended this new concept. "I wonder about jealousy."

"What about jealousy?" Dr. Best tried to follow her leap of thought.

"Preachers constantly say that everyone is guilty of the sin of jealousy. But I don't remember ever feeling jealous, at least not after high school. Did I not feel what was there, or wasn't jealousy there?"

Leaning forward, Dr. Best parried with a question. "Lily, isn't jealousy a distortion of the drive to enjoy the best that God put on Earth?"

"And eventually I didn't think I had a right to exist, much less enjoy anything. If I didn't have the right to enjoy things, then I wouldn't have been jealous. At least not consciously." Again there was silence in the room. Then Lily sighed deeply. "This is good. But, Dr. Best, I would never have understood any of this if I hadn't suffered so much."

"Now you understand what the Apostle Paul meant

by the merit of sharing the fellowship of Christ's suffering, Philippians 3:10."

"I wish I could tell every mentally ill person that his suffering doesn't have to be meaningless—that it can result in insight and knowledge the average person doesn't have-- that he needs to keep searching until he finds the truths deep under his illness. I wish I could tell every counselor that a person can be Christian and crazy. Emotional illness is not evilness."

"Lily, when you truly believe that, you can."

The following morning Lily dutifully reported to her last day on the unit at state hospital for the retarded. As she passed from the nurses' station into the resident's hallway, she heard a strange cry, "Eey-ah," and the pad of bare feet running toward her. A boy in institutional gray clothes, with pale skin and dark shaggy hair, ran right into her.

"Why, Stevie, you came to greet me! Hi there, baby!" Lily embraced the laughing child. "How did you know when to watch for me? I never will understand how you kids know things like that. I wonder what goes on inside your heads that you can't tell us about."

Tenderly Lily caressed the child's cheek and then, cupping her hands under his chin, turned his face to meet hers. "Say, Stevie, that old sore on your cheek is all healed. You must have stopped banging your face. You're a good bo-ey. But, oh, that snotty nose of yours. What a mess!"

Lily pulled a tissue from her jacket pocket and playfully dabbed at the boy's nose. She gazed deep into his Teddy Bear brown eyes and thought she saw a hint of a twinkle there. "Stevie, did anyone ever tell you that you have beautiful eyes? Well, you do, and you know what---I love you." Without stopping to look around, Lily planted a quick kiss on the child's forehead.

"Hey, you, what the—." Attendant Jamison's fat form had rounded the corner and was lumbering toward her. "What you think you doin' with that boy? He in breakfast line, then he gone."

"It's okay, Mrs. Jamison. Stevie came to say good morning to me. I will take him to breakfast."

"He supposed to be in line. He can't—"

"I said I would take him," Lily cut in sharply.

The startled attendant waddled off, mumbling, "Sure be glad when you gone, uppity lady."

Lily put her arm around the child's shoulder, guiding him toward the dining room. "Stevie, I'd be glad to be gone too, if it weren't for you and my other kids. Come on. Let's get some breakfast and have a good morning together. I'll get the others and we will all spend the day in the playroom." Stevie smiled and snuggled against her side.

Lily's plan for a happy day was shattered when, at 10:00 a.m., she heard herself being paged over the intercom. "Lily Farmer, come to the office for a staff meeting. Lily Farmer to the office."

In the office of the unit director, Lily heard the unexpected news that all residents under eighteen years old were to be transferred to a schoolhouse unit that day. Recent legislation required that all children be in classes taught by licensed teachers. Children listed as severely and profoundly retarded would be housed in Smith Hall, the former toilet training building, and they would attend classes and activities there, with a licensed teacher.

Lily's heart sank into her stomach. How could they do this to her children! Her leaving would be hard enough for them. To return them to what they had experienced as the toilet training building would devastate them. The attendants so often used Smith Hall as a threat. The residents would not understand that returning to Smith was suddenly a promotion. Was there anything she could do for them?

As she listened to plans for the transfer, Lily realized that the attendants would herd the children like cattle, never stopping to soothe or reassure them. Intentionally defying the system, Lily asked the unit director, "May I move my own therapy cases? If I walk over with them, they may be less frightened."

The director eyed her suspiciously. "Suit yourself. Just don't get in the way."

An hour later the herding began. Lily tried to stay ahead of the forced march, taking her cases from each ward before it was called. During the walk to Smith Hall, Lily put her arms around each child. "It's all right. You're going to a new home, a nice home. Smile." The children went peacefully enough into the Smith building, but Lily could tell from their eyes and the tension in their bodies that they were hurt and angry at what seemed a return to the hated toilet training.

Finally Stevie's ward was called to move. Since all the residents were under eighteen years old, the group of forty would move en masse. When Lily arrived at the ward door, Attendant Jamison had lined up the residents against the wall.

"What you want?" the attendant grunted. "I'm busy, and you stay away."

"I am taking Stevie myself." Without waiting for a reply, Lily took Stevie by the hand and hurried out. Finding a quiet alcove in the hall, she pulled the boy close to her and began talking reassuring to him. "I don't know how much of this you will understand, but I'm going to try. Stevie, you are going to a new home. A nice home." The twinkle that Lily had discovered earlier returned. "Right, Stevie, toys and a teacher. Games. Music." The child bounced on his bare toes. "Yes, Stevie, music. Now, listen closely. The new home is Smith Hall, but Smith is different now. No more toilet training. Smith is good now."

At the mention of Smith Hall, Stevie backed away from the therapist and tears welled up in his eyes. "Oh, Stevie, it's all right. Your new home will be fun." Stevie remained unconvinced. Lily drew him to her and hugged him and cooed. "It's all right, baby. It's okay. Be a good bo-ey. I have to take you to your new home."

Arm around the child's shoulders, Lily guided Stevie down the hall to the exit doors. As they left the building, spring sunshine poured over them, and Stevie gurgled happily. *Maybe this won't be so bad,* Lily thought.

In a few minutes the therapist and child stood at the doorway of Smith Hall. "Here we are, Stevie. Let's go in to your new home." Tears filled the child's enormous brown eyes again. "I'm sorry, little one. This has to be. I can't help you now, baby."

When an attendant appeared to unlock the door, Lily was pleased to see the elderly black lady whose help she had sought previously for Stevie. Blinking back her own tears, Lily pleaded, " Be good to him and he will respond."

"Miss Lily, I'm going to be on his ward all the time. You know I'll be good to him. Come on, Stevie."

With an agonizing yell, Stevie jerked away from Lily and ran through the doorway. On the other side, he turned around and, for the last time, Lily saw his face, mucus streaming from his nose, tears staining his red cheeks. With sudden anger he pounded his fist hard against his cheek and rushed wildly down the hall.

The door closed. Lily wept alone. Was her work all in vain? Would the new attendants be good to Stevie? Would he really have classes, or was this another token to satisfy the bureaucrats? She would never know.

That night, sitting cross-legged on her bed, her drapes open to let in the comforting moonlight, Lily picked up her journal and wrote: "Matthew 2:18, In Rama was there a voice heard…Rachel weeping for her children and would not be comforted because they are not.' Jesus, I weep for my children and especially for Stevie. Stevie is gone, and I will never see him again on Earth, never hold his bony hands in mine, never comfort him, and never stroke his cheek until he breaks into a smile. But though I cannot be with him, You can. Into Thy hands I commend his spirit. I will be comforted that someday I will see Stevie in Heaven, and he will be perfectly whole."

She stared out her window, sending her prayers for the children into the blue. Then she sighed, looked down at her journal, and started to write again. "I must press on, build a new life, and find a new job. Heavenly Father, Mighty One, I need Your strength to face the future." Lily bit her lip and blinked hard. "How can I look an employer straight in the eye, smile, and say, 'I can do the job,' when so often I haven't been able to do the job? I couldn't handle the fire and glass in the lab. I didn't fit with the teachers in the city. I was a total failure at state hospital. Do I need a new kind of job? One working with moral, middle-class, small town people in a nice setting. One with no messes or smells. Maybe a dorm counselor at a Bible college. Or a pencil pusher in a government bureaucracy.

"But, oh, Jesus, I would miss being with children. They are my friends, my love, and my lifeblood. What I really need isn't a new kind of job but a new me to cope with the job. Maybe the me that Warren, Lena, and Dr. Best seem to know. There must be something You can do." The heavens were silent. "Oh, well," she said aloud, "So much for wishes. I might as well read the book that Dr. Best assigned me."

Getting the small green book from the top of her dresser, Lily sat cross-legged on the blue-green plaid bedspread, opened the booklet, and resignedly scanned the first chapter. 'What a title," she mumbled. "Failure as Necessary for Spiritual Growth." She began to read aloud, " 'Oh wretched man that I am! Who shall deliver me from the body of this death?'" [Romans 7:24] Tears spilled from Lily's eyes. "God, that is how I feel. A body of death. I'm locked inside a body whose illness defeats everything I do. The next verse is thanking God that I'm rescued through Jesus Christ our Lord. But I can't thank Him. I've learned what it is to be identified with Christ's suffering and death. But I am still in the grave and can't find the resurrected life. "

Lily continued reading. Abruptly she sat up, alert, intrigued. "This book says that in fact I already have what I need: I just don't know it *in experience*. I already abide above with Jesus and reign with Him, in fact. I just need to experience what is already fact. The book gives a method for joining fact and experience. It says to find out what is fact. Then, even if I don't feel it, 'act as if' the fact is real to me, and eventually it will be. The key is 'act as if'. "

Getting up on her knees and turning toward the big window over her bed, Lily gazed at the bright moon through the budding maple branches. "The moon has no light of her own, but she's 'acted as if' she did, treating the sun's light as her own for so long that beholders see the 'as if' as fact. And I bet that if the moon could talk, she would say, 'Of course it is My Light. He, the Sun, gives it to me.'

"Can the Son give His Light to me? Does He already give His Light to me in fact, though I don't know it in experience? Can 'as if' create fact? Or the experience of fact?"

Lily sat back on her heels, watching the shifting moon shadows. "I wonder--. Is there a psychological parallel to the spiritual 'act as if' principle? Something to unite fact and feeling? Something like, if I act as though I am confident and competent, eventually I will become competent and confident? Because I already am. Or, if I act like I am free, then—." She caught her breath at the magnitude of the thought. "But is it fact that I am free?" She glanced at the open Bible on her dresser. "Yes, it says, 'If the Son therefore shall make you free, ye shall be free indeed.' {John 8:36] But will the principle work? Will it really make me free?"

Not daring to hope too much, Lily dropped down on the bed, turned off the table lamp, and whispered, "Please, Jesus, please make me free." Then remembering her decision to accept God's will, she added, "If the life of illness is Your will, then Your will be done." Lily slid under the blue-green quilt and fell into a restless sleep, the gentle moonlight guarding her dreams.

May 1974

Monday and Tuesday flew by as Lily hunted for a new job, but the door to secular employment had bolted itself. Either jobs required more stamina than Lily possessed or her qualifications did not fit the standard requirements. Besides job-hunting locally, Lily had previously mailed out inquiries about positions in Christian schools and missions. A month had passed with no responses. But, to her surprise, she was not particularly bothered about lack of employment. She was too intrigued by the changes going on within her.

When she met with Dr. Best for the sixth time, the psychiatrist began by asking, "How is the diet coming? Are you trying to avoid the foods on the list?"

"Yes, it is pretty easy, really."

"You have been working on this for four weeks. Do you see any difference?"

"I don't have the stomach aches or the headaches." Lily looked out the window at the rolling green lawn, listened to the robin in the hickory tree. " Vision and hearing are clearer, more dependable."

"What about mental symptoms?"

"I still have the hallucinations." She paused. "Now that I think of it, I don't get upset about them. The old irrationality does not take over often. I haven't had the overwhelming fear and anger for –hmm—for about a week. But I thought that was the psychological and spiritual progress. Is it a change in chemistry because of the diet?" she asked, brushing a loose curl out of her face.

"It is both. As your chemistry becomes more normal, your brain can function more effectively. Your senses function more accurately. Your thinking and emotions become more normal. So, you can use what you are learning spiritually and psychologically. Changing chemistry with diet or nutrients or medication does not change the problems that have built up over the years, but it makes it easier for you to solve them yourself. "

"I wonder—I mean, I like the change," Lily stammered. "And can we change subjects?" Dr. Best smiled and nodded assent. "I've been reading the booklet you assigned last week. It quoted Ephesians 2:6, God 'raised us up together, and made us sit together in heavenly places in Jesus Christ...' and another verse in Second Timothy 2:12, 'If we suffer, we shall also reign with Him...' So if we reign in heavenly places, we must be like royal sons and daughters, like princes and princesses. But my experience isn't about reigning: it is about failing." Dr. Best gestured that he was understanding. So Lily continued, "But, according to those verses, I must be royalty. Not because of any attribute of mine but because God says so. I learned a long time ago that what God says is Reality."

Dr. Best leaned back in his chair, hands folded as if in prayer, watching Lily closely. "Yes, what God says is Real. Now where are you going with this?"

"There is some principle that I can't quite grasp. I can't even clearly say what I am sensing. Some parallel between the spiritual and the psychological. It has to do with living according to fact, not experience. The spiritual fact of reigning with Christ is like the real, factual self psychologically. Spiritual feeling is like self-concept. My self-concept has been horrid."

Unexpectedly Lily caught her breath. The winds of the old illness howled through her head. Lily's composure trembled under their blast. She pressed her hands against her forehead.

"Dr. Best," she gasped. "Something is bothering my head. Something about my real world, my Island home. Division. Two self-concepts. Two worlds. A queen reigning. A guilty one hiding. Like the spiritual split. Shawn reigns. Lily suffers. Dr. Best, I'm losing you. Fog. You're too far away."

"Lily, you are all right. You are perfectly safe here. Tell me about Shawn. Tell me about your island."

Abruptly, Lily straightened in her chair, rigid, eyes locked forward, and recited without expression, mechanically, like a poorly memorized speech. "I am Shawn, queen of the Lone Palm Island. I live in America to gather information. I had not been on the Island for two years, but when I lost my job, I had nowhere else to go. I returned to my Island. Lily, my American disguise, is weak, a failure, guilty, condemned. I am competent, adequate, deserving respect. I can meet people, handle problems, and deal with life. Lily cannot. Lily gets hurt. I do not. I reign: Lily–"

The recitation stopped. The confession had penetrated her own mind, calling to her newfound self-respect. The Lily-part of her spoke slowly, intensely, "Dr. Best, that is it. The Lily-Shawn dichotomy. Like the dichotomy between how I act and what God says I am."

"Are you saying that there is a difference in who you really are and how you regard yourself?" the psychiatrist questioned.

"I'm not sure who I am. Shawn and Lily were never totally separate, not like in a multiple personality. They were both I; I would never have told anyone that my name was Shawn. They were just different frames of reference." She sighed and stared at her loafers. "But I lost who I really am between them."

"When do you remember first thinking of yourself as Shawn?"

Lily turned her eyes away from him and gazed at the corner of the ceiling. "Let's see," she said thoughtfully. "First grade, no. Second grade, third, fourth, no. Fifth grade, oh no!" Lily's body tensed to hold her in place. She gripped the arms of the chair to fight the impulse to run from the room, to hide her shame.

"It's all right, Lily. Look at me." With effort, Lily complied. "Now tell me about it. I accept what you are experiencing as valid." Dr. Best leaned forward, as though lending her his strength.

Lily spit out, "In fifth grade, the movie. Soldiers in India. Gold and silk swirling. Strange music. Spies. A child queen. The movie was real for me." Lily hung her head, feeling that she had irrevocably disgraced her world. "Oh, Dr. Best, my beautiful Island all started with a kid's Saturday matinee! A friend took me to a movie, and I got lost in it." Finally, after so many recitations, understanding of the origin of her internal world penetrated through all her defenses. There could be no more denial, no escape. For several minutes, Lily remained motionless, tears dropping profusely into her lap. Then she murmured sadly, "Now I have fully faced the truth: I have ruined my secret home."

"Not necessarily, Lily, your island is a lovely retreat." Lily's eyes flew wide open at the strange statement. Dr. Best continued, "It is like a dream castle. Great men have had dream castles. Because it had a childish beginning doesn't make it any less beautiful."

"You are not going to attack my Island?"

"No!" he said emphatically. "I am interested that you find the real Lily. Then the island will take care of itself."

Startled, Lily recalled hearing the same idea from Dr. Willoughby six years previously. With this shock, Lily's mood changed abruptly from shame to curiosity. "Find the real Lily? How? I keep changing back and forth."

"A few moments ago, you described Shawn as self-confident, capable, talented, deserving respect. She must have gained those qualities from her creator. The creation cannot be greater than the creator."

"I created Shawn," Lily said quickly, almost defensively. Then more cautiously, she asked, "Do you mean that things that Shawn is and can do are really my own?"

"Certainly. Wasn't Shawn simply a way of explaining to yourself feelings and experiences you did not understand? Wasn't the movie just a tangible experience of lostness in a world that confounded you?"

Lily mused, "That movie must have been about the Indian revolution against the British. I was fighting my own inner revolution and picked up the movie's feeling tone, without understanding it. I had rarely seen a movie, and the feeling of confusion generated by the strange sounds and motion embodied the confusion I already felt. When Shawn came to be, English was not her native language."

"Your way of accounting for your confusion about

words. The distortion of word meanings that you have struggled with is probably part of a basic brain dysfunction."

"Yes. And since I was already convinced that I was so different I couldn't be human, Shawn had a non-human ancestry. I understand." Lily's stony pallor melted into a shy smile. She was intrigued by her own discovery. "Shawn was simply an attempt to explain everything that confused me."

"Not so un-human after all, is it?" Dr. Best said. Lily laughed a little with her psychiatrist. "It is normal for a child to want to understand her world. I think you will find your island has lost its power over you."

Automatically defensive, Lily struck out, "The Island did not have power over me. I ruled it. It—." Then hearing her own recitation, she paused, grinned, and laughed nervously. "Yes, I guess it did. The Island kept me from knowing myself and from facing the world of people where I would get hurt."

A rose-soft peace descended on the room. Sunbeams filtering through the open draperies danced across the floor, over Lily's feet, and crept up her arms. A gentle silence rested on patient and doctor for several minutes as Lily allowed the new insights to penetrate all through her being.

Then, quietly, as though afraid the speaking would be the undoing, Lily murmured, "It is gone. The old tunnel of darkness." Dr. Best raised an eyebrow questioningly. "In college, I felt as though I were walking through a long black rubber tunnel suspended in the darkness of outer space. There was a light at the end and I kept hoping to reach it. The day I exploded at college and the university psychiatrist sent me back saying nothing was wrong, I reached the end of the tunnel. The light went out. I stepped into utter darkness, floating hopelessly. With Dr. Willoughby, I returned to the tunnel, hoping it would land on Earth. Just before we started this session, I saw myself in the tunnel reaching out of the end for a flower but instead I got sticky mud. You and I just removed the mud, the confusion.

"Dr. Best, I'm standing on solid ground in full sunlight. The tunnel is gone." Smiling, Lily raised her closed hand. "I hold my flower, an Easter Lily. Today is Resurrection."

"Praise God." Dr. Best said. "Be happy and thankful and rest this week. We'll talk more next Wednesday."

CHAPTER 28—SALVATION IN THIS WORLD
May 1974

Saturday morning, Lily awoke early and popped out of bed to see if her new world was still there. "Oh, those colors! Those gorgeous spring colors!" Lily exclaimed, leaning out her window and gazing across the yard.

For two entire days, Lily had marveled at what her senses were showing her, at the realness and stability of the physical world. No longer did objects appear flat, cartoon-like, shifting about at a whim; instead, the trees in the yard, the people on the street, the furniture in her room were a study in three-dimensional steadiness. Light and dark were clear, separate phenomena without fog or mist to blur them. But the most marvelous thing to Lily was the colors--each one pure, clear, individual--not splotched or smeared.

"Fantastic!" she said aloud to herself. "The grass is green—all green, not mixed with orange and blue. And, oh, those pink and white blossoms on the dogwoods! I'd forgotten they looked like that. And the sky is blue, bright blue, not lead gray. So many years since I've seen this. No wonder the Psalms sings the glory of Creation. Oh, Jesus, what a marvelous day! Now I've got to find just the right thing to wear."

Opening her closet, Lily ran her hand along the rack. She would be spending the whole day with her girlfriends from church, attending a seminar led by a well-known Biblical counselor. She wanted to wear something bright and dressy but also comfortable. "Perfect," she announced as she pulled out a leaf-green pantsuit and flowered blouse. "I'll look like I'm wearing spring."

A few minutes later she drove her red Chevy toward the church. *What is this going to be like, to go with the group as me, Lily? Two weeks ago I would have been terrified of exploding under the pressure of the unknown, and Shawn would have taken over. But now I can do everything Shawn did. How will it be to laugh and tease and sing, just like everyone else?"*

Promptly at 8:00 a.m., Lily steered her freshly washed car to the curb in front of the church. Staring at the group of young people gathered on the sidewalk, Lily gasped, "My goodness, they aren't cartoon flat any more. Yeah, there's Babs. I guess her car didn't get fixed." Lily rolled down her window. "Hey, girls," she called to her three friends near the curb. "Come on. Get in. My turn to drive."

A blonde girl in a stylish Hawaiian mu-mu opened the car door, laughing. "Hi, Lily! What's got into you? You never drive," Babs quipped as she and the other two girls got into the car.

"I'm blossoming," Lily laughed, indicating her flowered outfit, but in her own mind enjoying a much more significant meaning.

Soon Lily joined the caravan of cars on their way to a neighboring suburb where the meeting was being held. Her passengers bantered back and forth about clothes, hairdos, new fads, and summer plans. Previously, Lily would have thought this talk too frivolous and unspiritual and tried to direct the conversation toward the seminar. But today, the new Lily reveled in belonging and chattered right along with her friends.

However, after their group had arrived at the large, modern auditorium and found their reserved seats in the balcony, Lily began to question whether the day would continue to be so wonderful. The difficulty of orienting herself in an unfamiliar building and the noise of the milling crowd were causing the feeling of confusion she thought had gone forever. Would other symptoms reappear also? As she read through the printed program, she saw the subtopic, "The Sin of Anger", and her apprehension intensified. Silently, she prayed, *Jesus, I think I am into more than my newfound self is ready for. Help me harness the capability of the old Shawn to remain calm and steady.*

In spite of her efforts to sit still like her friends, Lily squirmed in her seat as the featured speaker launched into his first lecture. With charts, diagrams, and examples that ridiculed anyone different from himself, the lecturer expounded his own theory of human personality, dwelling primarily on its shortcomings and sins. *Another salesman type, full of fast-paced verbal garbage, but no depth,* thought Lily. *He could use a semester of Psych 101. And when is he going to get to the dynamic Christian living part. I need answers, not a sales pitch.* Lily crossed and re-crossed her legs, doodled on the program, and surveyed the faces of people she knew in the audience. *How can these people be so caught up in such a shallow presentation? Oh, well, maybe the next hour will be better.*

The next hour was worse. As Lily concentrated on controlling her irritation and refuting the speaker's negative view of human nature, she heard, "All anger is sin. I mean ALL anger. When I yell and lay on the horn in a traffic jam, that is a sin."

Lily boiled. *What is the matter with this guy? Number 1, why get so worked up about a traffic jam? Number 2, that's petty peevishness, and not real, solid anger. Number 3, anger is a gift, a healthy self-protective response. Paul said to be angry and sin not: deal with the situation and let go of it before night. This is the kind of prattle that almost destroyed me. Surely people from our church will know better than to believe this.*

Lily scanned the audience, picking out individuals that she or Warren had counseled. To her horror, each one seemed to be absorbing the speech uncritically. She wanted to scream, *No, you mustn't believe him. Rejecting anger will destroy you. Use anger; control it; but don't call it sin.*

Abruptly Lily noticed that people nearby were looking at her, that she was poised on the edge of her chair, muscles taut, fists clenched. She forced herself to sit back. *Jesus, help me be logical and calm. Maybe the speaker will clarify his statement later. It is only fair to give the man a chance.* The speaker offered several more examples of petty irritation as illustrating anger as sin, and then he moved on to denounce other normal emotions. Lily fought hard against her fidgeting. *Controlling this new me isn't easy. It would be easier to switch to my fantasy world and escape, but I'm determined to stay in reality.*

When the session ended and people approached the platform with questions, Lily threaded her way to the front of the auditorium. Just as she reached the steps leading to the stage, the speaker came down them. Lily called to him. "Excuse me, sir, would you clarify something for me?"

"I have time for one more short question before lunch," the speaker replied, glancing in her direction.

"You said all anger is sin," Lily began, working hard to keep her voice neutral. "The Apostle Paul said to be angry and sin not. When Jesus cleansed the Temple, He behaved angrily. Would you please correlate this with your statement that anger is sin?"

"Jesus was not angry. He had righteous indignation at the Jews' sin against God. He was not personally involved."

"Where do you draw the line between anger and righteous--." Before Lily had finished the question, the speaker had turned his back on her and walked away through a nearby door. Lily stood alone, dumbfounded that a noted speaker, a Christian leader, would be so abrupt. Then the old self-doubts assailed her. Was she overly-demanding or hostile? Was she too unimportant for the speaker to bother with? Was she...? Was she...?

Fighting back the tears, Lily rushed for the nearest ladies' room. Safely alone inside a stall, she allowed a few drops of liquid hurt to flow. "Dear Jesus," she whispered, "I need to talk to someone to get perspective." But lacking anyone to talk with, Lily pushed herself to analyze her own feelings. "I am angry because I believe that a lie was perpetrated -- because I think that people could be damaged by the lie--and because I feel personally insulted. Keep me calm on the outside until I can work through this on the inside."

With a pasted-on smile, Lily joined her friends outdoors on a blanket spread on the green lawn for a picnic lunch. Though she tried to be pleasant, she felt her agitation affecting the group. What should she do? To her delight, she spotted Warren propped up alone against a shade tree at the far end of the lawn. Quietly she excused herself and ran to him. She dropped down on the grass in front of him.

"Hey, Warren, I didn't know you were coming."

"I thought I might pick up a few pointers to use in counseling."

Lily gasped, "Warren, you wouldn't really use what this man said, would you? He contradicts everything I ever heard from you."

Warren scrutinized her closely. "You're upset, aren't you? What did the speaker say that got to you?"

"That anger is sin. Warren, you know as well as I do that anger is a normal, healthy God-given emotion."

"And I know a young lady whose anger is of a different nature than most people's."

"There are different kinds of anger?"

"Certainly. Anger from different sources and to different degrees. The anger many people have is a self-centered over-reaction to some minor, passing situation. Like a man yelling at his wife because she burned the meat."

"That's not really anger. That's peevishness."

"To many people, that is anger."

"That is not my anger."

"No, your anger recently is a reaction to what you see as unjust or harmful to yourself or another person."

"Right. And I try to use the energy from the anger to right the wrong."

"That kind of anger is what some Christian counselors call righteous indignation."

"It feels like anger to me!" Lily leaped up, hands on her slim hips. "What would you say about my old lake of rage? That came out in violence I could not control. That was anger in the ultimate. Are you going to tell me that it was sin?"

"Cool down, Lily. Your old rage was entirely different from the anger the speaker is talking about. That was a combination of chemistry and your past. Don't apply a principle unless it fits."

That evening, sitting cross-legged on her bed, Lily sorted through the day's experiences. In her journal, she wrote: "Maybe the difference in what is healthy and what is sinful is how nuts you are. What's healthy if you are nuts is sin if you are healthy. I guess I'm better off being nuts."

Early Monday morning, Lily bounded into the waiting room of Warren's counseling center. "Hi!" she greeted him as he stood beside the coffee pot. "Got any time for one of the proverbial 'angry young men' who happens to be a woman?"

Warren chuckled, picking up his coffee cup. "Sure. Are you still worked up over that seminar?"

"Only halfway?"

"Which half?" Warren settled on the well-used couch and gestured for Lily to take the overstuffed chair. She sat gingerly, avoiding the broken spring.

"I'm still worried that some people we know in the audience will believe that man and be hurt by what he said."

"Lily, I hate to tell you this, but you are wasting your energy on people who don't need it. I have watched those people listen to speaker after speaker and appear to accept every word. Two weeks later they have forgotten all that was said if it didn't fit into their own personality system. The people you are concerned about are already battling their own deep anger, and one more speaker won't make much difference. The worst thing that can happen from such lectures is that normal people will be convicted of their peevishness, as you call it. Then they might give others with deeper anger a hard time."

"And it is my job to counteract that hard time."

"Go to it, Lily. I don't know anyone better qualified for the job."

Lily heaved a sigh of relief and, grinning, got up, chose a red mug, and helped herself to the coffee. "Say, Warren, what are you doing today? Could you use some extra secretarial help?" Lily knew, and Warren knew, that she was looking for a place to be.

Warren said, "I don't need a secretary, but I could use a substitute counselor for emergencies while I am gone this morning. And this afternoon I have a session with the family of the girl you are working with. If you are available, I will ask them to bring the child too."

"Great. At least I'm useful for something."

Lily manned the counseling center not only that day but for the following two days until time for her appointment with Dr. Best. The experience of being "in charge" chased away the thunderclouds that had gathered in Lily's mind after the seminar.

By the time she reached Dr. Best's office, a new joy fairly bubbled up inside her. As she strolled across the court of the office mall leading to the psychiatrist's suite, she prayed, *Jesus, I wish life could always be this way— head clear, vision bright, limbs swinging free. I know it could be if only--."* If only what? Something in the back of her mind was pushing for recognition.

Lily paused by the fountain in the mall courtyard, watching the water spray high into the air, then fall back like thousands of tiny diamonds. Lily imagined the gems sinking down, down, and found herself admiring the mosaic at the bottom of the pool.

I used to say I was like a mosaic, made out of thousands of beautiful pieces, but I kept coming unglued. That's what's bothering my head. Jesus, I need emotional glue. Would You please show Dr. Best how to manufacture it? Thank you.

As confident as if she knew what to do in this therapy session, Lily tripped lightly into Dr. Best's office and was soon sitting in her usual chair facing him.

"How are you today, Lily?"

"Happy!" She laughed at the quizzical lift of the psychiatrist's eyebrows. "Really I am. I still have problems, but I'm happy in spite of them."

"I believe you are." A smile spread across Dr. Best's square, smooth face. "How was your week?"

"Thursday was hard. It was a week since I had to say good-bye to my children at the state hospital and I was worried about them. But I survived. Friday I was flying high because my whole world had been transformed. Dr. Best, you'll never know the joy of suddenly discovering a world of color, of dimension, of sound that is dependable, that doesn't change at every whim of circumstance." Lily noted his nod of comprehension.

"Anyway, Saturday I attended a lecture with our church group. The speaker was one of those overly aggressive salesman types who strike me the wrong way. I got a bit upset and for a while thought I would go to pieces like I used to. But, Dr. Best, I didn't! I talked to Warren, then got busy doing things at which I am competent. Instead of falling apart, I am stronger for the trial. That has *never* happened to me before."

Dr. Best beamed his approval. Then he asked, "Lily, was this the well-known speaker that I saw advertised on Christian television last week? The counselor who has a negative view about human nature and emotions."

"Yes. He made a major issue that all anger is sin. I'm glad that last week we talked about all emotions being God-given."

"If we had not, how do you think you would have reacted?"

"Guilty," Lily responded before she thought.

"Guilty?" Dr. Best had expected a response of anger or an answer involving the old psychotic symptoms. "Tell me about it."

"If I had heard him a month ago, I would have felt guilty. Guilty and condemned to be forever guilty on this Earth."

Dr. Best asked, "On this Earth?"

"I'm forgiven for eternity. I know I'm going to Heaven. But I'm always guilty of something here—saying the wrong thing, folding my socks the wrong way, having feelings different than other peoples. Always guilty of something." Overcome by a wave of memories, Lily hung her head. "There is no way out. Not here."

"Lily, you know that Jesus died to pay for your sins. You have asked him to save you from your sins." Dr. Best groped to understand Lily's dilemma.

"It is not just sins. It's all the guilts. They're too many, too strong. Too all present." A pained whine slipped into Lily's voice. She wrapped her arms around herself and stared at a spot on the beige carpet. Then, tearfully she said, "I'm sorry. You have helped me with past guilts so they don't seem so important. But there will always be new ones. How can I pay for them? Self-inflicted pain and verbal abuse don't work anymore. Even fire doesn't pay for them."

"That is right. You cannot pay for your guilts, real or imaginary. Even when you punish yourself, the guilts will still be there to be paid for again and again. Christ died on the cross to pay for those guilts once and for all."

"Even the imaginary ones?"

"*All guilt!*" Dr. Best spoke sharply. "As I said before, Jesus paid for all your guilt and guilts, even the neurotic ones. Accept His payment."

"But I am guilty of instability daily. I can't change that. I have tried."

"Lily, that is enough! Look up here," the psychiatrist commanded. She lifted her head, showing the face of a hurting child. But Dr. Best would not allow her to regress into the old pain. "Stop and think. Instability is a condition: it is not the basic you. Poor relationships with people, role confusions, inappropriate words, and so forth are *not* who you are, but what you do. God's power in you can help you change what you do—bring it up to who you are. You are a member of the family of the Creator of the universe. God the Father is your Father."

"But He is a judge." Lily protested. "A judge looks at obedience to the law. I can't understand all the laws about people, much less obey them." Before she could stop herself, the awful thing that stood between Lily and God the Father leaped out. "Don't you see, He has to punish me, like my father. I never know when I'm going to break a rule and get punished. So I punish myself first."

"Lily!" Dr. Best thundered. "GOD IS NOT LIKE YOUR FATHER."

"But the Bible says that God the Father judges our guilt."

Dr. Best looked away for a moment, and Lily had the impression that he was praying. Then in a patient, firm voice, he said, "Lily, that is not God's kind of judgment. Maybe this story will help. Once there were two friends who completed law school together. One became a highly successful judge, known for impartial and severe sentences." Lily nodded and looked out the window toward the sky, picturing the scenario. "The other lost his money, his job, and his self-respect."

Under her breath, she whispered, "Me."

"One day, the righteous judge looked down from his bench to see a dejected man in tattered clothes. The man accused of many crimes was his old friend. The evidence was indisputable. The just judge had no choice but to pronounce a sentence of guilty. Gazing straight into the criminal's eyes, he handed down the full penalty of the law–$50,000 fine or ten years in prison. But the judge was sick at heart as he looked at his old friend, knowing that the man could not pay the fine and probably would die if imprisoned. In an unexpected move, the judge stepped down from the bench. From under his black robes, he pulled a checkbook and wrote out a personal check for $50,000, all he had in his account. 'Here,' he said to his old friend. 'The law demands justice; my love for you demands mercy. Pay your fine. Then come home and stay with my family.' Lily, you can accept or reject Christ's payment for your guilts-- all of them, past and future, known and unknown, within your control or out of your control. The choice is yours, right now. Decide! Will you accept His payment, and NEVER try to pay for them again?"

Lily struggled. She had accepted Christ's payment of sins sufficient to enter Heaven. Now she was asked to accept His payment for her on this Earth, to let go of the lifelong self-chastisement. To take from Him with no possibility of giving in return. She struggled for several minutes. Before her closed eyes appeared a picture of Jesus reaching out His hand to her. How He would hurt if she rejected His offer! Gulping down her false pride, her lifelong insistence on giving rather than taking, she took a deep breath and said firmly, "Jesus, I accept. I will let You pay for my guilts, even the ones I cannot stop because they are false feelings in my head. Thank you."

"Jesus says your penalty is paid." Dr. Best pronounced it as a final verdict.

"I am forgiven?"

"Forever. Forgiven forever and decreed to be righteous."

"Righteous? Having a right to be?" The words permeated all the way through Lily's being. A profound relief rippled through her body. It seemed too good to be real. She looked to Dr. Best for confirmation. "Not because of anything I have done or can do, but because He says so?" Dr. Best smiled and nodded authoritatively. "It's too much. It takes the responsibility off of me and puts it on Him. He has the strength for it. I don't, but He does."

"Exactly. That strength and love given to us is called grace. You know the verse, 'By grace are you saved....' "

"Saved from the old illness? Saved from my self? Salvation in this world. If that is true, it means I can someday be free."

"Then, Lily, be free."

After that session's unexpected ending, Lily encountered one surprise after another. With awe, she noticed that she respected, even liked, herself. She was surprised at her own strength and resilience. Even the appearance of old symptoms could not shake her newfound freedom. One day as she worked in the yard, enjoying the spring sunshine, her vision began clouding. For a moment she saw tiny white squiggles drop from the sky. A surge of self-condemnation threatened.

"Oh, no, brain, you can't fool me. I won't fall for your tricks. I like me. Why not? God does." She clipped a long sprig off the forsythia bush. "Besides," she laughed. "How many people have built-in picture tubes?"

CHAPTER 29—FREEDOM
May 1974

"Lena! Lena! It came!" Lily shouted, slamming through the front door and running into the kitchen, waving a piece of paper over her head. "The letter from the mission school. It came."

"Slow down and tell me what you are talking about." Lena turned around and, laughing, leaned against the kitchen cabinet.

Lily took a deep breath and held out the letter to her older friend. "You know I applied to teach in several mission schools. I've been accepted at a children's home and school in the Appalachian Mountains. The letter just came. Here."

Lena took the letter and read the first paragraph. "It says you are *tentatively accepted* as a special education teacher."

"I have to go down there soon for an interview and a short trial period. I'm not worried. They need a *licensed* special education teacher, and those are hard to find. I'll going to be a missionary—really—truly—finally. Like I always thought God wanted me to be."

"I'm glad for you," Lena said, turning toward the stove where she was cooking Friday's supper.

"What's the matter," Lily asked. "You don't look glad."

"There's only three weeks before you have to leave. I'll miss you."

"I'll miss you too. And all my friends here," Lily said, bouncing on her toes. "But I'm not going to the ends of the earth. I'll be home frequently. And you can even come and see me. Isn't that town near where you grew up?"

"About seventy-five miles, as the crow flies," Lena said slowly. Then focusing on Lily's joy, Lena turned to her with a smile and a laugh. "I'm being silly. You've been wanting to do something like this. Let's celebrate! I'll make your favorite strawberry cake."

"Oh, thank you." Lily flung her arms around Lena in a big hug. "Now, I've got to call Babs. And Warren. And my pastor and– Oh, no!" Lily exclaimed. "How am I going to get there?"

"I guess you'll drive that red car of yours," Lena chuckled.

"By myself? There's no way. It's five hundred miles. I could never see well enough to drive that far."

"Oh, Lily," Lena chided. "If God wants you to go, there will be a way. Stop worrying. Now, go call your friends. I have to get busy. Cakes don't bake themselves."

After supper, Lily, Lena, and Lena's ten-year-old daughter sat around the table, reminiscing about their two years together. Lena, who rarely talked about herself, shared life in the mountains as she remembered it from childhood. Then she asked casually, "What did your parents say when you told them about the job?"

"Uh—Um, I haven't talked to them," Lily said sheepishly.

"You—what! Lily, they are the first people you should have told."

"Uh, do I have to?" she said with a sideways grimace. "What if they don't want me to go? You know how my mother can be."

"Of all the--. Do you believe this is God's will for you? Or don't you?"

"Yeess, but–"

"No buts! You go call them right now," Lena commanded. "I'll sit here and pray."

Reluctantly Lily got up and took the cordless phone from the desk to her bedroom. A few minutes later, she emerged, all smiles. "Whew! That's over. They were okay. They even seemed happy. My father wants me to come home in the morning so we can talk about it."

"And are you going to go see them pouting and expecting trouble? Or are you going to trust God to work things out?"

"Uh, trust God?"

"Yes! If He wants you at that school, He will work out the details. Now let's pray and go to bed."

*****

Sunday evening, Lily's red Chevy zoomed into Lena's driveway, horn honking. Lily jumped out and ran around the house to where Lena was weeding the flowerbed, shouting, "You were right! You were right! He did it!"

Lena sat down at the picnic table. "By *He,* you mean God?"

"Yes, God worked it all out."

"Oh course He did. Now slow down and tell me what happened with your parents."

"At first, I was scared that they would say *yes* but put all kinds of obstacles in my way-- as usual. They didn't! I showed them the letter and the brochure about the school. My father hugged me and told me he was proud of me. My mother got all teary eyes and then asked if I needed her to make any new clothes to take with me. That's the biggest offer she could make. And--." Lily plopped down on the bench across from Lena.

"And what?"

"You'll never guess. My parents are going to help me drive to the school. My father is taking vacation days from work. He will drive their big car and Mother will help me drive mine. He got out the maps and we figured out the route—roads, rest stops, and all. My father even said we are staying in a motel overnight—two nights if I 'm getting too tired. *My father* who never stops once he is in a car."

"See, Lily, when you give them a chance to do something they are capable of, they show that they love you. You just have to let them do it their own way."

"Lena, they want me to go, even after I told them I won't be paid enough money to live on and will have to use my savings. They even volunteered to help with expenses!"

"What did you expect? Honestly, for a girl who says she knows Jesus personally, you seem to keep forgetting--."

"I know. God will take care of it." Lily put her hands on her hips and announced with a mischievous grin, "Some times I think He might actually like me, not just have to put up with me because He's God. Maybe even my parents like me a little."

"Or maybe you are beginning to like them a little. Has it dawned on you that you should accept your parents for who they are? Just as they are, without trying to change them?"

"Ouch!" Lily paused in thought, and then said, "That's what Prof Filbert told me eight years ago."

"Then it's about time that you do it," Lena chuckled.

"I get the point, and –" Jumping up from the bench, Lily grabbed up some yard tools and trotted toward the back door, calling over her shoulder, "Let's celebrate. I brought candy apple ice cream. And I'm starved."

By Thursday evening, Lily's excitement had been replaced by frustrations and doubts. As she sat on the carpet in her bedroom, boxing up papers and trinkets, Lena came in and sat on the bed. "You look upset. What is the matter?" Lena asked.

"Sacrifice!"

"Sacrifice?"

"Missionaries are supposed to sacrifice to follow God's call. But I don't have anything to sacrifice. No job. No home. No goals to give up."

"Do you think God is bothered about that?"

"Maybe. No, I guess not. But I don't like even the word. It makes my mouth taste bitter." Lena waited quietly for Lily to continue. "My parents were always sacrificing.

When I was little, my mother sewed for people to help with our income. When she sewed for the missionaries, she did not charge them. I'd see them drive away in expensive cars, when we didn't have a car. My father supplied mission groups with expensive tools when we needed the money to live on. Sometimes those people didn't even say 'thank you.' In college, I gave my money to foreign missionaries only to watch the kids of those missionaries spending money freely for things I could never afford." Lily slammed a stack of books into a box.

"What else?" Lena prompted.

"In chapel, speakers used to say 'sacrifice yourself on the altar.' I sacrificed and lost my self."

"Was that what God wanted you to do?"

"No, I know that now. But I still don't know what He does want. What does the Bible mean in Matthew 16 when it says 'If any man will come after me, let him deny himself, and take up his cross, and follow me'? I just don't know." Lily ran packing tape across the top of a box and marked it *Appalachian Mission School*.

"Didn't you tell me that the theme of your church retreat this weekend is 'Giving your all'? Maybe the retreat will help."

"Maybe."

*****

Two days later, on a chilly May evening, Lily joined her church friends at the retreat in an old converted barn, hidden away in acres of green woods now dripping wet after a spring downpour. As the twelve young people huddled around the fireplace to ward off the dampness, Lily felt a connectedness that she had never known during the four years she had been in the group. She stared into the fire crackling brightly, casting its yellow glow on the guitarist who leaned against the stone mantle. He strummed the first chords, and the group joined in, singing the familiar words, "We are one in the Spirit, we are one in the

Lord. And they'll know we are Christians by our love." The music took Lily back to that special evening at the Catholic college when the nuns had included her as one with them. Her heart soared. *We are one,* she thought, *All of us that love You, Jesus. No matter what our church, our group. We are one in Your love. One in Your joy. One in Your peace.* She glanced up at a spider that had been spinning a web in the corner. *It is so peaceful here in Your presence that no creature needs to be afraid. Not even a spider. Not even a fragile Lily.*

Gradually Lily realized that since that day of the affirmation of her true self—what she called "Resurrection"—not once had she been inundated by the objectless fear which for so many years had controlled her life. Since she had understood that she was adopted into God's family, since she had realized that she did not need to pretend to be a queen, that she truly reigned with Christ—since then, she no longer cringed at the ravages of this Earth but faced them confident of her own integrity, her own preciousness. When Reality had become real to Lily, pretense was no longer necessary.

The singing stopped as the pastor, a serious-faced middle-aged man, walked up to the fireplace and took his Bible from the mantle. His opening words startled Lily. "It is no accident that there are exactly twelve of you here tonight. Our group has been together for several years, but this is the last time we will ever meet. Two of you are going west to work on an Indian reservation. Two are going to teach in a Christian school in the Deep South. Lily is called to a mission in Appalachia where her family's roots were generations ago. Perhaps this is Christ's night to prepare all of us for a sacrificial ministry, as Jesus prepared the Twelve Disciples when He appeared to them in the upper room after His resurrection. The original Twelve were hidden behind locked doors, out of sight of the world just as we are. Suddenly Jesus was in the room with them, saying, 'Peace be unto you: as my Father hath sent me, even so send I you.' Then He breathed on them and said,

'Receive ye the Holy Ghost....' [John 20: 21-22] It is obvious that the Holy Spirit is here with us tonight, getting us ready for whatever lies ahead. The Spirit has given each of us special gifts but often we don't recognize them. I want us to help each other be aware of the gifts God has given us before we go out into ministry.

"One way to recognize our gifts is through the eyes of other Christians, by affirming in each other what you admire, what you see as unique. Right now, I want you to pair up, counting off by twos. Affirm in your partner the qualities which you believe that God can use."

Lily cringed. This sounded too much like the encounter group in her Human Development class years ago. She had grown since them, but would the result be the same?

The pastor was continuing. "Stay with whomever is your partner, even if you don't know that person well, and let the Holy Spirit direct you."

Lily stifled a groan as she realized that her partner would be one of the most popular women in the group, a well-to-do will-o-the-wisp whom she could not possibly understand. But obedient to the pastor's directions, she smiled as the girl reached out a hand in friendship.

Looking somewhat bemused, her partner suggested, "Let's pray for the Spirit's leading."

As they prayed, Lily felt a warmth, a new love for this girl who had had all the world's advantages that Lily had wished for. Then, at her partner's insistence, Lily began the affirmations. To her own surprise, she heard herself say, "Over the years I've watched you and wondered about you. You are so vivacious, so constantly happy, that I found it hard to relate to you. I am thankful for tonight to overcome my resentment. Your most outstanding qualities are your energy and enthusiasm. You are always bubbling, smiling, and cheerful, with a ready quip and a light-hearted love for everyone. God can certainly use you in a ministry of cheer."

To Lily's amazement, her partner stared at the floor.

"Lily, I'm not what I seem to be. I don't know you well enough to affirm all that God has done in you. Your intelligence is obvious. But what I admire is your straightforwardness, your honesty about yourself. You say what you mean. You are different."

Tears welled up in Lily's eyes at the mention of the hated word with such power to hurt. "Yeah, I'm different. I always have been."

Her partner interrupted. "But don't you see. You know how to be honest, transparently honest. No hypocrisy. No pretense. You don't have to wear a mask." The girl halted, her voice dropping in dejection. "I wear many." Lily gasped in surprise, groping for words to help her partner.

Unfortunately, at that moment, the pastor stood up to make announcements, cutting off their time for serious sharing. Immediately, Lily reacted with frustration, her old anger threatening to burst into flames. But just as quickly, the anger died, and Lily slipped into the happy mood of the group. During the supper hour, Lily chatted with her friends, describing the mission school to which she was going, sharing in their plans, joining in the laughter and fun. Even the mention of her difference had not disturbed her sense of belongingness.

At 8:00 p.m., the pastor called the group to the fireside chairs for evening meditation. He began, "Our theme tonight is Matthew 16: 24, 'If any man will come after me, let him deny himself, and take up his cross, and follow me.' The call to self-denial has sounded through the centuries of the Christian church, but in our modern society of conveniences, we have forgotten the meaning of sacrificing ourselves...."

Lily's whole being rose up sharply in protest. Powered by her newly gained health, she shouted in her innermost being, *No, no! I just found my self. I will not deny it. I will not sacrifice my self. I am. I will not say that I am not. I will not return to naquan, to non-entity. I claim all my own feelings, my thoughts, my essence, and my right to be. I will not be extinguished.*

The pastor's words were lost as haunting voices of past authorities reverberated in Lily's head. "Make your bed with square corners." "When you leave food on your plate, think of the starving children overseas and feel ashamed." "Good Christians never get angry." "Avoid boys and worldly amusements, and lest they tempt you, stay ignorant of them." "Pray three times a day and read your Bible twice." "Guitar music is the instrument of the devil." "Put yourself last and others first."

Lily closed her eyes, and toward all the legalistic captors of her childhood, she hurled her missile. *Jesus said, Know the Truth and the Truth will set you free. I know who I am, and you cannot bind me to the image of a model child any longer. I will not be confined by ignorance and narrow mindedness. I will know about the world; I am not so weak that knowledge presupposes my entrapment. I will enjoy life, and be thankful to God who made that enjoyment possible. I will take care of myself, because if I don't, how can I take care of anyone else? Judges of the world, I like me just as God made me. And if you don't, that's your problem.*

The haunting specters of Lily's past scattered to the far corners of the barn and disappeared forever. Never again would she be chained to the old illness. Opening her eyes, Lily rocked back on two legs of her chair and folded her arms in satisfaction. *Pastor just said, "Be transformed by the renewing of your mind." Thanks to Jesus, I have been. No more volcano. No more Island. No more tunnel. No more need to escape. I am Lily, and I am free.*

www.ingramcontent.com/pod-product-compliance
Lightning Source LLC
Chambersburg PA
CBHW071157240526
45470CB00016BA/192